EAT THIS BOOK

The Last Diet Book

By Billi Gordon

So what if your muumuu is so tight you can see your heart beat. Just keep laughing. Eventually you're bound to lose some weight, and if you don't ...

A WEST GRAPHICS PUBLICATION

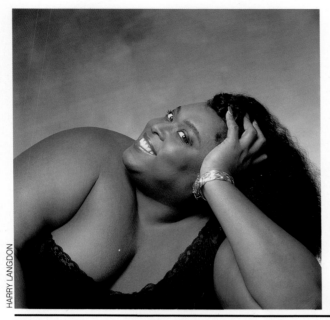

HARRY LANGDON

About The Author

Billi Gordon, a University of Michigan alumna, was born on a dirt street called Tuthill Road, across from the city dump, on the wrong side of the small blue collar town of Dowagiac, Michigan. Growing up across the street from the city dump, she naturally grew up to be trash. (But when men of position, wealth, and breeding see trash, they pick it up—and that has been Billi's salvation.)

Currently, Billi sells more greeting cards than any other model in the world, and with nearly one hundred hit greeting cards on the international market, she is the undisputed and unrivaled queen of character modeling, earning her forever the encomium "Le Mannequin Extraordinaire."

As well as being an internationally reknowned model, Billi is also the author of the best-selling, humorous cookbook, *You've Had Worse Things In Your Mouth*, which *The Saturday Review* hailed as, "the humor classic of 1985."

Billi spends her leisure time talking to her agent on the telephone or cocktailing at expensive hotels while discussing the stock market with all the businessmen she used to "know" before she became a successful actress, author, poet, television writer and model.

© 1987 by West Graphics
R. West Productions, Inc.
576 Natoma Street
San Francisco, California 94103

Printed in Japan

ISBN 0-9614979-1-2

2 3 4 5 6 7 8 9 10 edition

ART DIRECTOR
R. West

EDITOR
Randall Weischedel

TYPOGRAPHY / DESIGN / EDITOR
Augustus Ginnochio

PHOTOGRAPHY
John Edwards (unless otherwise noted)

□ CONTENTS

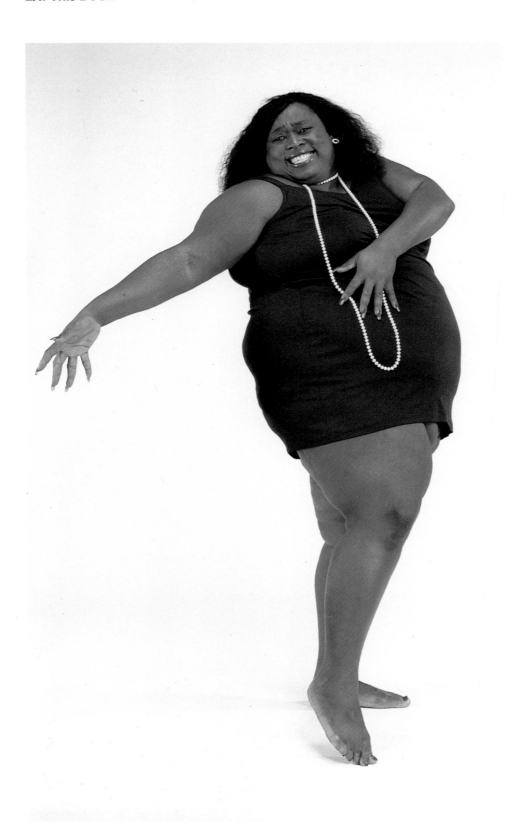

These hips are my credentials.

☐ INTRODUCTION

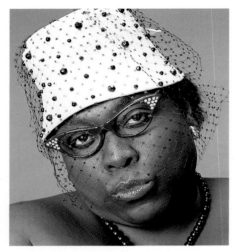

Why, one might ask, would 475 pounds of dark, sweet, abundant womanthang, such as moi, write a diet book—of all things? Especially since everyone knows I've made my statement by being endlessly luscious, and I've even managed to pay the rent along the way. So, what's in a diet book for me? Truth, honey! It is about time that somebody who is truly qualified gives a testimonial regarding the rigors of dieting and its supposed rewards.

Now, who writes all the diet books today; skinny, little, white heifers in designer leotards, with tortillas for tits and protein powder on their breath. Most of them have only lost five pounds in their entire lives, twenty at the max. In all due respect, what these girls know about dieting is as valuable as what Princess Di knows about breakdancing. It's the woman who could fall down on the street and rock herself to sleep trying to get back up who's the expert—not the girl who could walk through a harp. It's the woman who the city tried to wrap in gauze and run through the tunnels in order to clean them out, who's the real pro, not the woman who when she turns sideways and sticks out her tongue looks like a zipper.

Yet, day after day, year after year, it goes on; these skinny heifers sitting up there writing book after book, on diet after diet, talking out of their boney behinds, smelling up this good world. Well, I'm here to put a stop to this poppycock, cause as Queen Victoria would have said "we are *not* amused", or you know how they say "the opera ain't over till the fat lady sings." Well, I'm about to sing, honey.

I have divided *Eat This Book* into several basic sections: *Diets, Powders, Plans & Scams*—The only diet; *Low Calorie Dishes, Weight Nazis* and *Give Me Linguini or Give Me Death*.

One section, *Diets, Powders, Plans and Scams* deals with all of the various diets that are out there to try and why you shouldn't waste your money, time or effort. In this section I give the simple facts about how to go about losing weight easily and scientifically. At the end of that section you will find the beginning of my calorie count list which will just give you the calories of some everyday food items.

Another section, *Low Calorie Dishes* is some simple recipes that are low calorie, if you so choose to trouble yourself by going out of your way to make *Diet Food*. At the end of this section, the calorie guide continues.

A third section, *Weight Nazis*, is a section that deals with a frontier that most diet books don't deal with, and it is *fat bigots*. It deals with the people who think they have the right to call you Noah's Ark as you saunter through an airport lobby, and the rednecks who put the "No Fat Chicks" bumper stickers on their trucks. This section will teach you how to create utter chaos in an airport without being arrested by the FBI for interfering with the Federal Aeronautics Regulations and will also teach the simple technique of turning over pick-up trucks without chipping your nailpolish.

Give Me Linguini or Give Me Death is a section that is pretty self-explanatory. It is for the girl who does not want to lose weight, and who has chosen to believe the old saying, "Nothing wants a bone but a dog and he don't want it if he can get some meat." It is for those many heavy-hipped women, who if the truth were told, prefer Big Mac's to Proposals, and Twinkies to dates. In short, this chapter is another new frontier in diet books, how not to diet successfully.

Speaking of new frontiers, I have developed a whole new technique and theory in weight reduction. It's based on applying the myth to your everyday life ... you know the myth, the myth that fat people are jolly (tell it to Quasimoto). That's right, the theory is called laughersize; you're bound to burn off caloreis if you just keep laughing. So what, if when you started putting on your pantyhose Madame Butterfly was a caterpillar. Just keep laughing. So what, if your muumuu is so tight you can see your heart beat. Just keep laughing. Eventually you're bound to lose some weight, and if you don't ... just keep laughing!

On that note, in the name of abundancehood, and on behalf of the Sisters of Plenty, I give you *Eat This Book* ...   ■

☐ DIETS, POWDERS, PLANS & SCAMS

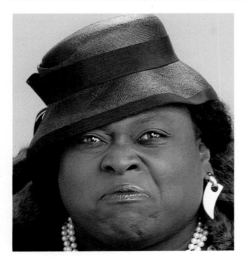

If I had a dollar for every diet I've been on, honey, I could afford to buy myself a waist, my girlfriend Maxine a set of hips, and my friend Cynthia a pair of tits that didn't point towards Australia. There's the water diet, the weekend diet, the cow urine injection diet, the high protein diet, the carbohydrate diet, the yogurt diet, the granola diet, the protein powder diet, and the fruit diet. That about covers the ones I've tried this month. Yes, and there are more exercise programs than there are pointed-toed shoes in Spanish Harlem.

Not to mention that there's enough instant weight-off "miracle pills" on the market to make Orca fit in Flipper's panties, if these cures worked. Of course they don't, and so as some sleazy, polyester suit-wearing, greased-back, receding hairlined, baggy-lipped fool laughs his way to the bank with the money from some fat girl who was foolish or desperate enough to believe his ad, another fat girl goes to the mail box anxiously looking for her gravity belt or her purse size gym.

Enough already! If there were as much good lovin' around as there are diets and diet plans, most of us wouldn't be overweight. And do you know what's the great irony about all this? Losing weight is as simple as birth control, you just close a different orifice ... i.e. your mouth. The formula is very simple.

Take it from a girl who has been hypnotized, acupunctured, injected, wired shut, strung out on diet pills, enemaed to death, and even had her refrigerator chained and locked shut—losing weight is very simple. All you do is you weigh yourself, multiply your weight by ten, and that is the number of calories, roughly speaking, that it takes to maintain your present weight. So in order to lose weight, merely eat fewer calories than it takes to maintain your weight. Now how easy is that? It's as simple as one of the Mandrell Sisters. You don't need any elaborate plans, and though some foods are harder to digest than others, supposedly causing some calories to be easier to burn off, that's a myth. To your body a calorie is a calorie, very much like to moi; a sailor is a sailor, and it's all in a day's work, honey. You can eat anything you want and lose weight as long as you don't exceed the amount of calories it takes to maintain your weight. Of course if you have metabolism problems this might not hold true for you. However, for most of us, (like 99%), these are the simple facts or, as I would say, "That's the 't', honey."

Now, if you genuinely want to lose weight, I have included a relatively comprehensive calorie guide for today's womanthang. It has everything from sushi to sperm with all the in-betweens. If you really want to lose weight, this guide, the knowledge of your present weight, and a willingness to count calories every day are all you need. ■

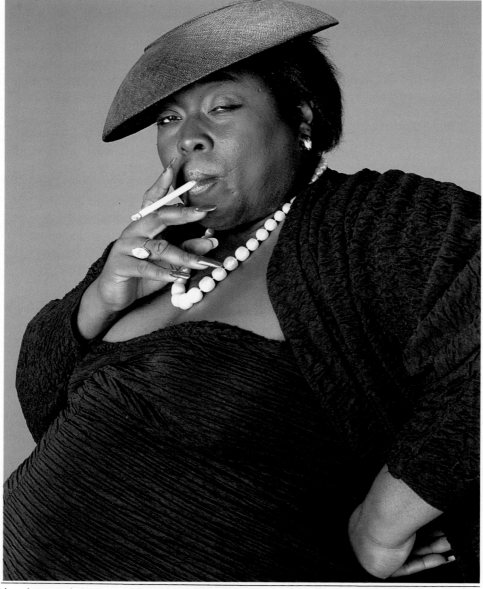

Losing weight is as simple as birth control, you just close a different orifice.

☐ GIVE ME LINGUINI OR GIVE ME DEATH

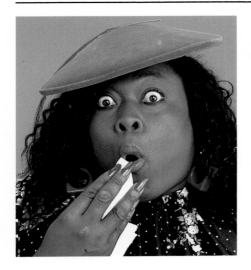

And what if I don't want to be skinny? That's right, you heard me Flo. So don't flare your nostrils at me and start flappin' your gums about never being able to be too skinny or too rich. I say, lies and garbage! I've seen some heifers who look like their necks are blowing bubbles, and when they walk their bones rattle so much it sounds like two skeletons breeding on a tin roof. But that's not the point. That's their cross to bear or not to bear. We all have to drag our own crosses down that Via Delorosa and listen to that wood banging on that cobblestone, picking those splinters out of our backs, those thorns digging into our foreheads, for one reason or another.

As I did in my first book with Revenge Cooking, it is time for me to break new ground in this arena. This time the new ground is how *not* to diet successfully. Everybody and their emaciated mammies have written diet and exercise books, invented gyms, pills, plans and powders that will show you how to get rid of your luscious hips, but nobody has told you what to do if you really, deep down inside, away from the intimidation of the crowd, don't want to lose weight. So my dear, I, the NAP (Negro American Princess) will teach you how to not diet successfully.

First of all, my precious Sister of Plenty, ask yourself this question: Why do I want to lose weight? Do you want to lose weight because you are genuinely unhappy with yourself and you don't like the way you look? This is not to be confused with what you've come to believe by conditioning. If you feel that your health is threatened, and this is a major concern to you, fine. If you are uncomfortable because you're overweight, which is not to be confused with being made uncomfortable by weight bigots, then fine. But if you want to lose weight because your friends or lovers are hounding you, forget it! Or because you don't have any friends or lovers and you're convinced that losing weight will change that, forget it again, honey. If that's the case you might as well be trying to get George Bush on the cover of *Jet.* You must free yourself, Sister of Plenty, and let the hips fall where they may!

■ Step 1:
Letting Farrah Go

In this marvelous, sexist, primitive, racist, ageist, self-destructing society of ours there is a little belief that the ultimate expression of beauty is a tall, athletic, youthful, Nordic blond. Granted, Malibu Ken and Cheerleader Barbie are cute in their own right, but they hardly hold the monopoly on beauty. It's like saying orchids are the most beautiful flowers there are, and then going on to claim that the beauty of a rose is limited and diminished when specifically compared to the orchid. Lies! Yet we do say that to ourselves every day, in our TV commercials, beauty contests, and the many other theaters of the absurd that we indulge in. So, naturally a full figured girl, not to mention a brunette or a colored girl, is going to feel a might mussed after a few years of this bull-ticky.

However, the good thing about this gross injustice is that it's all a myth and the bottom line is you're only as pretty as you feel. As trite as that may sound, that's how true it is. So honey, just get up one morning and look in the mirror and say, "Mornin' world—a diva is born!"

You see, what happens is the fat girl gets the green weenie, so to speak. The skinny blondes get to wear all of the spikes and hot clothes and what do we get? Floral muumuus and earth shoes. Well, of *course* the men are going to find the skinny girls more sexy if they're sitting up there in mesh hose and leather mini-skirts and we're sitting there in maroon caftans and industrial pumps!

Go for what you know, honey. There ain't no law (and I'm surprised there isn't) that says a fat girl has to dress like a Franciscan nun on vacation. Who told you you weren't sexy? Society. And what do they know? They haven't got anything right about any group as of yet, so why should they start with Sisters of Plenty?

I say, if you got it, honey, shake it and show it. That's right, shimmy honey! Shimmy like there's a passle of Pollocks doing the polka in your Paw Paw Patch. You got to let these men know that there's a whole lot of chicken in the barn, and that they need to hurry up and come on over. Now, the only way to do that is to make sure there is a whole lot of shakin' going on.

Dressing in drab colors is not going to make a size 50 waist look like a 26. A fifty is a fifty, whether it's in a muumuu or a fish tail homewreckin' dress.

It is all in the attitude.

■ Step 2:
Dispelling the Myths

A s is the case with any oppressed group, the Sisters of Plenty are laden with several myths: 1. Fat is ugly 2. Fat people are lazy 3. Fat people are stupid 4. Fat people are sexually inferior.

It is our duty to struggle to dispell these myths. First of all there are a lot of things that are uglier in this world than fat. Not to mention that fat is only ugly because somebody told us it was ugly. Just like somebody told us that black was not beautiful. Fat is ugly if you make it ugly. It's just like a picture. You can take any picture and put it in the right frame and hang it on the right wall and it'll raise the eyebrow of every passerby. But if you treat yourself like a pail of wolf labia, you're gonna look like a pail of wolf labia.

It is also our responsibility to be as intelligent as we possibly can. This world is no Club Med and honey, even blondes can't afford to be dumb anymore. It may be the early bird who gets the worm, but it's the wise old owl that's keeping it.

Now, as far as sexually inferior goes, this is the fun one to dispell. A long time ago I remember my mother standing in front of the mirror in her purple pumps with the rhinestones on the toes, and she was giving the neighbor-lady some advice. It seems the neighbor-lady's husband was having an affair. Mamma said, "Don't worry, girl, if the booty is good, he'll be back" and with that, mamma sent the grieving housewife on her way. When the woman was out the back door, her husband stepped out of mamma's closet and said, "You're absolutely right, I'm back." So take a lesson from mamma.

Another myth is that "Fat girls have to be nice." Lies! Fat girls may have to be nice, but Sisters of Plenty do not have to be nice, Sisters of Plenty have to be good in bed. That's right, honey, let's get down to basics.

Number 1: Be a good womanthang. Honey, a Sister of Plenty should be able to suck a cantalope through the eye of a sewing needle. There's only one way to be able to do that. Practice. You might wonder where you will find someone to practice on. If you run into difficulty you just go up to a random young man and say, "Look, honey, it's only five minutes out of your life, but it'll mean the world to me."

Number 2: Learn how to use what you got, to do what he wants. Case in point: most men just want to be satisfied and leave your boudoir feeling good. Become familiar with your body, learn its assets and its liabilities, learn to use them both to work in your favor. Women of plenty are soft. Soft is sensual. Women of plenty are warm. Women of plenty can mold to most forms readily. Learn to be warm, soft, and abundant. Teach him how to love it, and the next time he sees another woman of plenty he'll know what's in store. Understand, sugar?

Now, as far as fat people being lazy . . . I can't help you with that.   ■

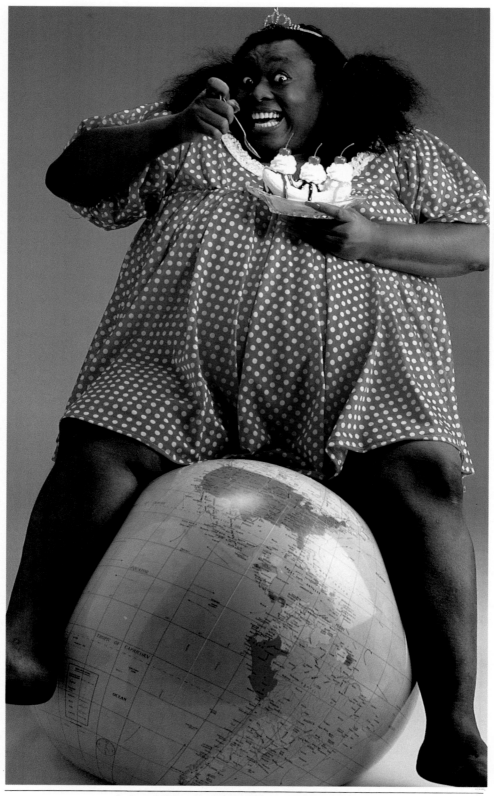

At last I found a diet that understands me.

□ DIET DISHES

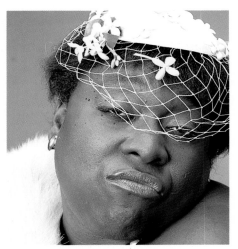

Well, if you ask me, every dish is a diet dish, it just depends on what your diet is. Nonetheless, a great many white heifers stricken by the diet craze go to great lengths to invent all types of ingenious diet dishes. And knowing the mentality of you girls out there, I just know if I didn't include some delectable, low-calorie dishes you would feel like you weren't getting your money's worth. Although I must admit you aren't registering that complaint with your husband, and God knows he's not giving you your money's worth, if he was, you would not have time to read this book.

As usual, I have the need to divide my dishes up into special sections. I mean, after all, a meal is not just a meal. There are different meals for different occasions. Now, I have divided this section into "Everyday Dishes," "I Need A Man Dishes," "I'm Gonna Eat That Man Right Out of My Hair Dishes," "Nothin' Wants A Bone But A Dog Dishes," and "I'm In The Grips of Grief Dishes."

I feel these categories cover the reasons we generally sit down to the table to eat . . . if the truth were told. However, I'm learning more and more as I grow older that the only thing we can count on to tell the truth these days are cameras and little children and little children can be bribed and photographs can be airbrushed. Is that God's way of telling us there ain't no such thing as truth?

I think it is. And I think it's just like my friend, Sam, the old wino who hung out at the corner of Six Mile and Woodward, in Detroit, used to say, "The truth only hurts for a minute!" And like my big sister Kate used to say, "Why would anybody bother themselves over anything that only hurt for a minute?" My big sister Kate was so wise. I miss her terribly. She's been a jail matron in India now for many years. Well, enough about truth and more about this section of the book.

Like I said in the opening, every dish is a diet dish, it just depends what diet you're on, and what you're using it for. For example, if one ate a barbecued sparerib, my friend Yuliis, who is as boney as the floor of a fish cannery, would say in her thick Norwegian accent, "Oh, daht's terrible! All daht red meat. It vill take it two years chust to get out of your system! It's very fattening and very bad for you." I maintain, however, that not only could they reshoot "Around the World in Eighty Days" with the excess hot air in her head, but that a barbecued sparerib, in the right instance, could be a diet dish. And that instance is: when it does not exceed the amount of calories you are allotted for one day.

□ EVERYDAY DISHES

■ LYNN KATHERINE

As is her namesake, this little heifer is full of surprises, and not nearly as white as she appears to be. She's simple, too ... the dish I mean.

1 head of Cauliflower	1 tbs. of low calorie Margarine
1 dash of Pepper	1/2 cup of Milk

All you do is take a head of cauliflower and break it into flowerettes. Put her in a vegetable steamer and steam her drawers off for about 20 minutes, or until she is real tender. Then you take her out and put her in a large mixing bowl. Add the milk and the pepper and the margarine.

Beat the girl with an electric mixer until she's as smooth as my agent. She'll taste just like mashed potatoes, but not with nearly the calories or the starch.

I'm really proud of myself for coming up with this dish, 'cause black folks don't eat cauliflower. You see, if it don't grow in Detroit, we don't eat it.

■ JOANELLA PYNE

If you don't like the taste of it, you can always throw it in your husband's face when he ruffles your feathers.

1 Rutabaga	1 dash Pepper
2 Turnips	1 dash Salt
5 Carrots	2 ounces Sour Cream
1 tbs. Dill	

Steam the vegetables until they are well done, then mash them. Add the sour cream (which, by the way is only 60 calories an ounce) and the herbs and spices.

Blend them very well on the high speed of your mixer until they are very smooth. Then put the mixture in the refrigerator and let it chill for at least 24 hours. It makes a wonderful nosh or spread for hors d'ouevres.

■ TESS ANN

As far as simple goes, this dish is second only to a Playboy Bunny.

1 cup of fresh chopped Kale	1/4 cup of chopped Onions
1 cup of fresh Collard Greens	

All you have to do is take the vegetables and put them in a bamboo steamer and steam them for three minutes. It's great. It's the latest thing in soul food. Soul food-Health food. It's called Sealth food.

The greens are quite good and have virtually no calories—and be great for your bowels.

■ DEADRA

Of course this doesn't look that dietetic, until you get done and see that proportion-wise it's enough food for two people. When you total up the calories in this dish and divide it by two, honey, you have Atilla's IQ.

8 ounces Turbot
1/2 cup of Bread Crumbs
2 tbs Bay Shrimp
2 tbs Imitation Crab

1/2 cup Low-Fat Milk
1 Egg
1/2 tsp Basil
Salt
Pepper

And speaking of quick and easy ... this is how you prepare it. First, take the bread crumbs and put them in a bowl. Add the milk, the egg, the basil, the shrimp, and salt and pepper to your taste. Stir this mixture until it forms a nice stuffing consistency.

Mold it to the shape of the turbot fillet and place it in a pan. Then add 1/2 cup of water and cook covered on high heat, until the water cooks away.

Oh yeah, I almost forgot the best part. Take the crab and place it tastefully over the top of the turbot. When this little sister is done, honey ... honey, hush.

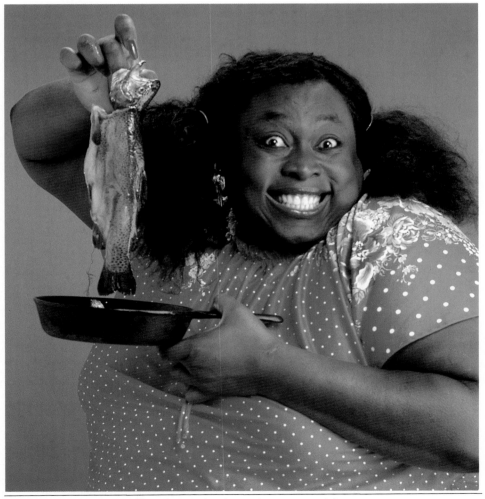

Feed your brain—starve your hips.

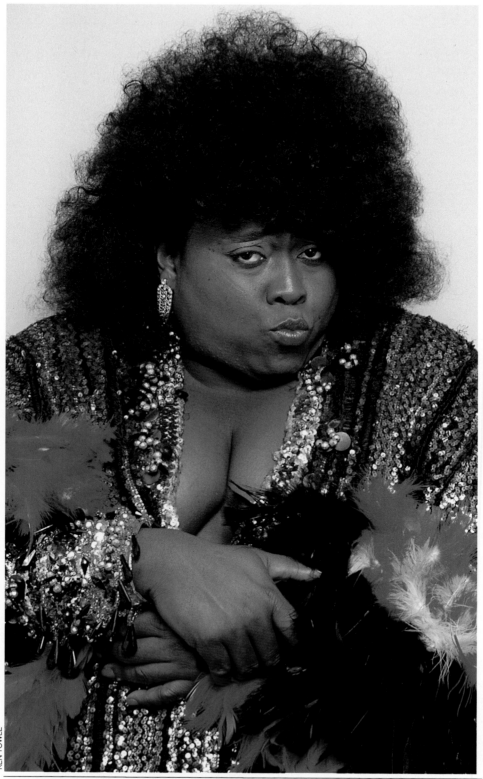

KEN TOWLE

*If you're not sinking your teeth into him tonight, it might as well be
one of these dishes.*

□ I'M GONNA EAT THAT MAN RIGHT OUT OF MY HAIR DISHES

■ BAWANDA BETH PEREZ

Now let's face facts: a good man, when translated, means a no good man, 'cause the good ones ain't no good, 'cause they don't have to be. Take a second and let that sentence sink in. Okay. Now back to facing those facts ... honey, when your man has done something in five minutes that affects five years of your life, you are not in the mood for carrot sticks.

Nor should you be. You need something to sink your teeth into, and since it ain't gonna be him tonight, it might as well be my wonderful chili recipe.

1 large can Chili Beans	2 lbs ground Turkey
3 tbs Chili Powder	16 ounces Tomato Sauce
1 cup diced Celery	1 can Light Beer
1 cup diced Onions	5 shots Tequila
	Salt

Take the ground turkey, onions and celery and brown them in a large kettle. Be careful not to let the turkey stick to the kettle. Ground turkey has virtually no fat, so you might have to add a tad of water to keep it from sticking. When the turkey is cooked and the vegetables are semi-soft (I'm sure you know that state), pour in the chili powder, then the beans, then the tomato sauce and the beer. Let this simmer for an hour and while it's simmering, knock off those shots of tequila and when he does come home ... you'll be ready.

■ JOSEPHINE BARBARINO

1 lb ground Turkey	1 cup finely diced Celery
1 can Tomato Paste	1 ground Bay Leaf
1 large Bell Pepper	1 tsp Basil
1 large Bermuda Onion	1 smidgen Salt
	1 tadlette Pepper

This is a dish developed from personal experience, honey. Years ago, when I was in college, I met a little blonde man of no particular excellence in any category. But for some reason I fell in love with him. It lasted about as long as college romances do. But I couldn't let it go at that. For years, I drug around the heartbreak of this man. I was dragging that cross down the Via Dolorosa listening to that wood banging on the cobblestones, honey—my lips long, my eyes tight, my head hanging low.

And ten years, and God only knows how many men later, this guy calls me up on the phone and says he and his wife are having their first baby, and you would've thought I was having it. But that's just how love be's sometimes—not how it is, but how it be's. It's like a palsy, like a flux, it just won't let go.

So this helped me. Brown a pound of ground turkey in a skillet, along with a finely diced bell pepper, onion, and cup of celery. Add the basil, bay leaf, salt and pepper. When the meat is brown add the tomato paste, mix thoroughly, and when the tomato paste is hot, go for it.

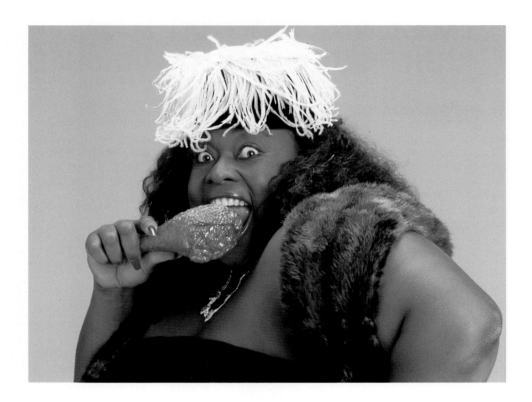

■ BELINDA CANTRINI

Belinda Cantrini will do what welfare won't.

2 fresh Turkey Legs
1 cup Flour
1 Egg
1/2 cup Skim Milk

1 tadlette Salt
1 smidgen Pepper
1 tad Poultry Seasoning

I advise saving this girl for times of true heartache. Like for example the time you decide to be Glenda Good Nooky and clean out your old man's car for him. After you've polished his spoked hubcaps with a toothbrush you start on the interior, and what to you find? A tampon! And you've just gone through menopause.

On a grave day like that is when you break out Belinda Cantrini!

First take two fresh turkey legs and bring them to a boil in a pot of hot water. After they reach a boil turn them down and let them simmer for about an hour.

While they are simmering you sift one tadlette of salt, one smidgen of pepper, one tad of poultry seasoning and one cup of flour into a bowl.

After that you beat one egg into one quarter cup of skim milk. Add this mixture to the sifted mixture. Then go over to the brandy cabinet and have yourself a shot of peach schnapps, sister, you deserve it.

After you've had a little schnapps and blended the flour mixture together well, you spoon it into the boiling hot turkey water. It makes wonderful turkey dumplings.

Let the dumplings cook on low in the pot for fifteen minutes. Then get out your address book and find a girlfriend that you really don't like. Take youself up a big helping of Belinda Cantrini, grab that fifth of peach schnapps and call up that unlucky sister to cry and smack in her ear all afternoon long.

■ JOSIE MAE

Five minutes alone with this dish and you will forget all about that no good man.

1 average package Spaghetti
1 can Campbell's Cream of
  Spinach Soup

8 oz. Natural Jack Cheese
1 tbs Vegetable Oil
1 cup Skim Milk

Into a pot of boiling water, imagine that you are putting the man who has worked your final nerve like it was the crossword puzzle in the morning paper. Instead of putting in this chump, put in the tablespoon of oil and then the spaghetti.

While the spaghetti is cooking, grate the jack cheese. Mix the milk and the cream of spinach soup together until they are well blended. Add the cheese to the mixture.

I know this may seem unnecessarily tedious, but I'm trying to give you something to do to occupy your frenetic energy and keep you from going out and choking some man to death and being sentenced to three to five in the local House of Corrections.

When the spaghetti is cooked. (You can tell by throwing it against the wall—if it sticks, it's ready . . . kinda like a hillbilly white girl.) Anyway, when it's ready, drain the spaghetti, and then mix in the cheese mixture and cook on a low heat until the cheese is melted. Stir constantly so the dish doesn't stick and so you achieve a smooth blended consistency.

■ NITTY GRITTY

1 pound fresh Green Beans
2 smoked Ham Hocks

3 large White Potatos
1 Bermuda Onion

That's right, honey, let's get right on down, as they say, to the Nitty Gritty. I don't know about the Nit, but the Grit part of the situation is, in most cases, caused by heartache; though the man was no good, he had a saving grace. And you knew he was no good from the start, but you got a hold of that saving grace. It was that saving grace that kept you pressing on, even though you knew mind readers were charging him half price and bald lesbian barbers were selling him hair restorer. You just kept holding on to that saving grace . . . so to speak. And now that he's gone the real issue is not the personal affronts or the social disgrace, or even the credit card bills; no, the real issue is no more saving grace.

So that's why I'm teaching you how to make this wonderful little dietetic gem. Take the ham hock and boil it in a pot of water until the ham starts to fall off the hock and the water is good and greasy. Throw in the green beans and the onion and let them cook for about 15 minutes, then throw in the potatoes and let it cook until the potatoes are done. Sugar, shucks!

Take yourself up a big helping of these green beans, white potatoes and hocks and honey, you will have found another "saving grace."

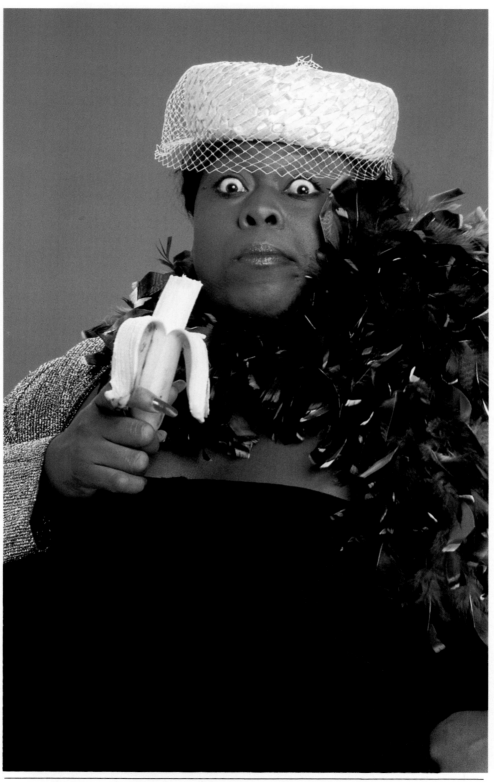

A kiss on the hand may be quite continental, but bananas are a girl's best friend.

□ NOTHING WANTS A BONE BUT A DOG DISHES

■ BERNICE

Have yourself a piece of this and tell me which one you like better, this pie, or the man last night? So hold office, Bernice!

3 large Sweet Potatoes	1 tbs Molasses
1 cup Cream	3 Eggs
1 cup Sugar	1 tsp Vanilla
1 tbs Honey	4 tbs Butter
	1 single Pie Crust

It may be an old saying, but honey, it's true, these men like meat—even though their wives don't know about it. They be calling me up on the phone saying, "Hello, heap o' mamma, is you is, or is you ain't my baby, now?" Yes they do, child. And you know why? It's not just because I'm shade in the summer and heat in the winter ... it's because where most girls have a straight highway, big mamma's got a scenic route.

Now back to the issue at hand. Take the sweet potatoes and boil them in a pot of water, until they are mashable like white potatoes.

While they are boiling, have yourself a little nip of Sambucca. (You never know when you're gonna run into an Italian man, and when you do it never hurts to have Sambucca on your breath). Anyway, cream the butter into the sugar, then you blend in the honey and the molasses, pull your chest forward, and say "Ouhhh" (it's just good practice) then beat the vanilla, the eggs, and the cream together. Add this to the sugar mixture and blend until very smooth. In a separate bowl mash the sweet potatoes and blend the sweet potatoes into the butter mixture with an electric mixer. Beat until it has a smooth, creamy texture (like my skin).

Pour this mixture into the pie crust and bake at 375 degrees until the crust is brown around the outside.

■ EDWINA WILLETTE

Honey, if Eve had known about this dish, she would've barbecued that rib that Adam gave her and had this dish for dessert.

5 large ripe bananas	1½ cups shredded Coconut
5 Eggs	2 tbs Corn Starch
2 cups Sugar	1 tsp Vanilla Extract
1 cup Cream	Vanilla Wafers
1 cup Butter	

Cream the sugar into the butter. Mix the eggs, cornstarch, cream and vanilla, and blend well. Blend the bananas and coconut into the butter mixture. Make sure the bananas are blended in smoothly.

Combine the two mixtures and cook in a double boiler on low heat until it thickens to a pudding consistency. Line a glass pan with vanilla wafers, pour the mixture, then put vanilla wafers on top.

Chill this for at least eight hours and tell your lips to prepare themselves to smack.

■ MARY LOU

Like any Mary Lou, this dish is a little on the cheap and plain side, but it's just too good to be ignored.

3 Turkey legs
1 can Cream of Mushroom soup
1 cup diced Mushrooms
2 cups cooked Rice

2 cups Milk
1 cup chopped Onions
1 cup chopped Celery
1/2 cup diced Pimientos

Take the turkey legs and boil them in a pot of water. While they are boiling on low heat simmer the diced mushrooms, onions, celery and pimientos in the milk and mushroom soup. When the turkey is done and tender, pick it from the bone and put it in the mushroom sauce mixture.

Then pour the whole thing over the rice and warm on low heat until everything is nice and warm and tender and good.. Just like you . . . right?

■ ROWEENA JACKSON

Keep this, not gloss, on your lips, honey child.

1 package Butter Beans
2 fresh Ham Hocks

1 small Onion

Boil the hocks, the butter beans and the onions until the butter beans are done. They will be very creamy and the onion will seem to have disappeared. De-bone the hocks and eat this girl like a WASP would eat bean soup.

■ DORIS

In order to get the true effect and best results of this dish, you have to put a tacky outfit on your back (anything from the sixties will do), get a surly, self-righteous look on your face (known as "attitude") and invite a big fat man over for . . .

12 large Green Tomatoes
1 lb. Bacon Fat

large bowl of White Corn Meal
Salt

Anyway, you cut the tomatoes up into horizontal slices about 1/8″ thick, then you salt them lightly. After that, you roll the tomatoes in corn meal. Meanwhile, you're heating the bacon fat in a skillet on the stove. When the bacon fat is hot, you slap those breaded tomato steaks into it, and fry them until they are about two shades lighter than Diana Ross. And ummm-mmmph.

□ **GRIPS OF GRIEF DISHES**

■ **QUEEN ESTHER HILL**

As complicated as this dish may appear to be on the outside, she's just all too simple to make, really, kinda like your basic Jewish girl ... to make this dish all it really takes is money.

8 ounces Crab Meat	1/4 cup Sour Cream
8 ounces Bay Shrimp	1/4 cup Miracle Whip
8 ounces Lobster	1/2 tsp Dill
1/2 cup finely diced Celery	1/2 tsp Pepper
1/2 cup finely diced Onion	1/4 tsp Salt
1/2 cup finely diced Radishes	1/4 tsp chopped Green Onions
1/4 cup finely diced Olives	3 cups cooked Seashell Macaroni

After you have cooked the seashell macaroni, blend in the sour cream and the Miracle Whip. (And I don't care how white you are, or if you can trace your family tree back to when they lived in it, DON'T substitute mayonnaise for Miracle Whip!) Make sure that it is blended in smoothly.

Then all you do is add the other ingredients one by one making sure to save the spices for last. To make this dish come out right, be sure to do two things.

First, make sure you find a large enough container so you have room to stir. Making this dish in too small a container is like a man getting romantic with a Sister of Plenty in a twin bed. Too much energy is lost keeping it off the floor.

Second, let this marinate all night (24 hours), and then eat it. Ummmmmm!!

■ **LI'L SUZIE**

Honey, go down to unemployment with this dripping out of the corner of your mouth and you'll get your benefits.

1 cup White Corn Meal	1 tbs Baking Powder
1 cup Flour	1/2 cup Margarine
2 tbs Sugar	2 Eggs
1 tbs Molasses	1 cup Milk

This is a recipe for when you're really in the grips of grief, like the time you got yourself fired because you fell asleep at your desk smoking a Virginia Slim (because you'd come a long way) and you burned up all the bookkeeping records for the past three fiscal years. Yes, hard times are at your door.

So nothing helps make hard times easier than some good corn bread and honey, this is a good corn bread recipe.

Now, what you do is you put on some Bessie Smith. Then you combine the dry ingredients in a large mixing bowl. Cut the shortening in. (If you don't have a pastry blender, two switch blades will do fine.) Beat the eggs, milk and molasses together.

Then mix this with the other ingredients. Blend until it is real smooth. Pour this heavenly mixture into a well-greased pan and bake it in the oven at 400 degrees for about 20 to 30 minutes.

■ MISS ACKLEY

1 cup Sour Cream
2 cups cooked Linguini
4 tbs Black Caviar

8 large cooked Shrimp, diced
3 tbs chopped Green Onions
2 Anchovies

You start by throwing the anchovies in the trash. Then take that trash and throw it on the doorstep of the person who is giving you grief.

When you get back home take the linguini and put it in a large bowl, then mix in the sour cream. Add the green onion and blend thoroughly.

Take the shrimp and throw it in . . . now, now . . . don't nibble, you need every grain of this recipe.

This is the hard part. (I know you've heard that before. Well, this time it really is.) Take the caviar and sprinkle it lightly on the top. Be careful not to let it clump together too much.

Let this dish stand and marinate for twenty-four hours. Just before you serve it, mix in the caviar.

Now hear this. If you decide to get cute, and mix in the caviar before you let it marinate . . . you know what will happen?

The fishy taste of the caviar will dominate the whole, entire dish, the shrimp might just as well have been carp, and you'll be even more in the grips of grief than you were to start with.

■ LOS SONAMBULA

This is for when you're *truly* in the grips of grief. This is not something to be used lightly for those everyday tragedies, like heartache, illness, death and despair.

1 fifth 151 Rum
1 large Pineapple, scooped out
3 oz Coconut Juice
3 oz Guava Juice

3 oz Mango Nectar
3 oz Kiwi Fruit Juice
3 oz Orange Juice
A lot of ice

Honey, save this one for when Golden Girls gets cancelled. Save this one for when Phyllis Schaffly becomes the first lady. This is one for when Jerry Falwell becomes President.

Take all the fruit juices and the liquor and mix them in a large container.

Fill the hollowed out pineapple with ice and pour the mixture over the ice. Find yourself a sturdy corrosion proof straw and a good palm tree and sit down and start singin' the blues.

(If you can't find a palm tree then I guess an oak or a maple will just have to do.) Confidentially, if you can't find a palm tree I'd double the proportions of rum.

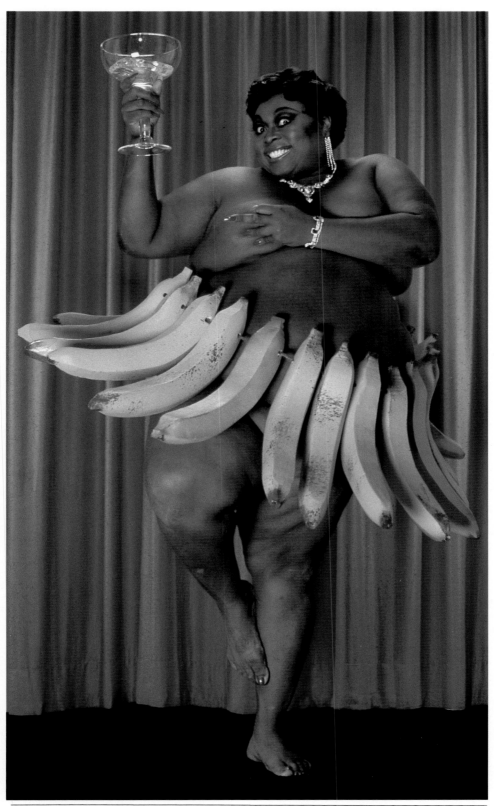

Trust me, this fruit is better on your lips than on your hips.

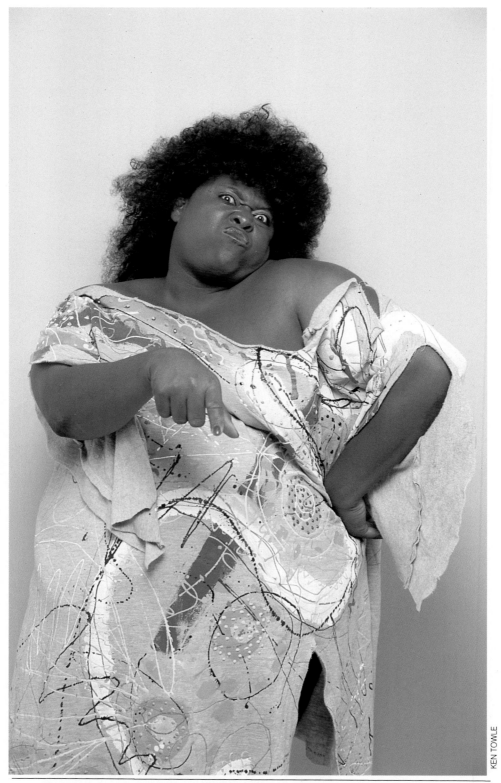

KEN TOWLE

Show me a weight-nazi, and I'll show you an anal retentive, closet vegetarian.

☐ WEIGHT NAZIS

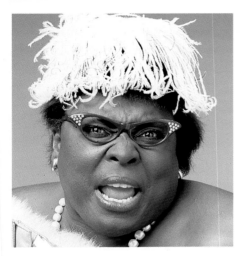

He walks among us, a low necked, drop-chinned, tight-lipped, sway-backed, fish-eyed fool. Yes and he's tackier than Persian decor, cruder than a Mexican dyke, he's the fat bigot, the hip hater ... yes he's the Weight Nazi. And what's worse, his bigotry and persecution is totally accepted. It's as legitimate as Florence Henderson to openly discriminate against and persecute fat people in this world today. Well, I am here to testify on behalf of the Sisters of Plenty: this must stop.

Weight Nazis are everywhere. Some of them dare to encapsulate their ignorance and put it on the bumper stickers of their pick-up trucks and Dodge Darts. I'm sure you've seen the bumper stickers ... "No Fat Chicks". Where do these suckers get off? There are a lot of things in this world, some things you like and some things you don't. However, I think it should be pretty obvious that you just take what you like and walk on by what you don't. Do I care about the sexual proclivities of some dimestore version of Hugh Hefner in a Chevelle? I don't happen to like men with small penises but you don't see me running around with a bumper sticker that says, "No PTMs" (Prince Tiny Meat). No I just sort through the crowd for the keepers and throw back the weepers.

You see it's all a part of the big male machine to oppress the Sisters of Plenty. That's right, honey. If you let these no-good men have their way they'll have you sitting up in some suburb doing time, wearing a tennis outfit, raising children and feeding dogs, with a stalk of celery hanging from your mouth. And just where are they while you're busting your breasts? That's right, sitting up there in front of the TV snorin' and pootin' like a fat Panda in a pea patch. Why? Cause while you were at the table eating sprouts and steamed carrots, he was smacking his lips on one of your great Italian dishes talking about how he wants to be buried in your linguini and embalmed with the clam sauce. And that's the 't' honey.

The whole thing is a big scam. These men sit up here and eat everything from stewardesses to waffles and get fat, bald, impotent, and everything else. But you let a girl get one little extra chin and he's ready to cut her head off and piss in her neck. I say it's time to fight back and take a lesson from Divorce Court, honey.

You see these white women aerobicizing and jogging and juicing and fasting and teasing, tossing, tinting, padding, pinning, and plucking trying to look good, and for what ... some man out there in the street spending your good mink money on the "bimbo du jour?"

Now, these same misguided, beguiled Suburban Suzies would have you believe that dieting is also an issue of discipline, and it's good to be disciplined. True, perhaps, but I done had most of their husbands, and not one of them asked me for any discipline. As a matter of fact I ain't never heard a man ask a womanthang for discipline—if you know what I mean. And if you don't know what I mean, honey, you never will.

Anyway, back to Weight Nazis. Weight Nazis must be stamped out in this society at all costs. A Sister of Plenty has an obligation to abundancehood to stamp out a Weight Nazi on sight.

Case in Point: I encountered a Weight Nazi down at the unemployment office a few months back when I was a Democrat. What happened was they had lost my claim, and my refrigerator looked like the Sinai on a windy day. So I had to have my funds immediately. After hours of waiting in a line that looked like the road to Juarez, I finally got up to the window and this ugly heifer, stood there looking like a teaspoon full of gnat labia. And you know there ain't nothing meaner than a ugly woman working a civil service job. There was enough space between this woman's teeth to hold a Polish Wedding. Her nostrils looked like the tunnel to Jersey. I kid you not. Kissing this woman must have been like parking in a two car garage. You know, it's amazing that when that woman bent over her lungs didn't fall out.

That heifer stood up there looking like, "So this is what happened to Haiti" and said, "Can I help you?" So I said "Yeah, cover your face when you're in public." You know that ugly heifer had the nerve to get offended. She sat up there looking like Bangladesh and flared those wide nostrils at me. Child, her eyelids were tighter than a middle class Jew in a recession, and they just went to twitchin' with bureaucratic attitude. Just about that time a gust of wind busted through the employment office and honey, don't you know, that heifer's hair did not move, but her neck did. It was not a pretty sight.

She asked me again if she could help me. I told her that I needed to get my unemployment check early because of some extenuating circumstances. That mongoose had the audacity to ask, "What's the nature of these circumstances?" I said traumatic. She said that was not sufficient information, and that she'd have to fill out a 34B. I said, "So get some silicone honey." She got mad, child. Yes she did .... called me thunder thighs! I slapped my hands on my hips, threw my head back and told that skinny, tight-eyed creekin' that I was gonna beat her till her tampon cried. You know, she had the nerve to say that I oughta get a job with the recreation department and let them fill up my navel with water so under-privileged children would have some place to swim. Can you believe the putrid gall of that troll? I told that back alley concubine that she looked like a cancelled five cent stamp, and that I was ready to throw her in the trash where she belonged.

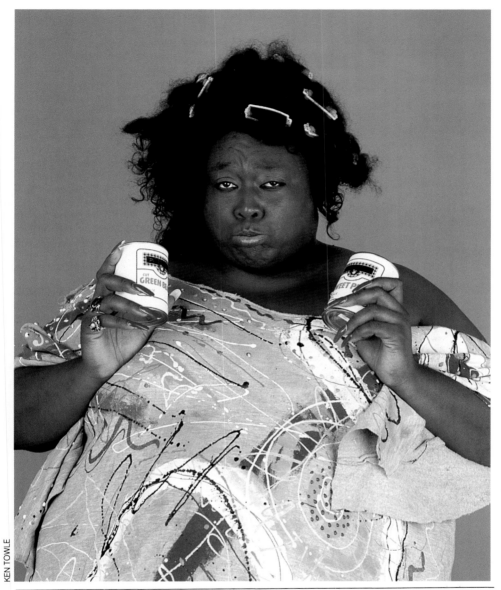

KEN TOWLE

. . . and then there is the poverty diet, (eat whatever you steal).

We got to tussling . I beat that heifer like she was a rented rug. I went up one side of her and down the other. I threw her down on the floor and did some break dancing on her neck. Honey, I whopped a knot on that heifer's drawers. And that's the way you have to deal with these Weight Nazis. Just jump right up in their face and slam dance, honey. This might not change their attitude towards the Sisters of Plenty but it certainly will change their behavior. And let's face it, it's their behavior that's giving us the flux! ■

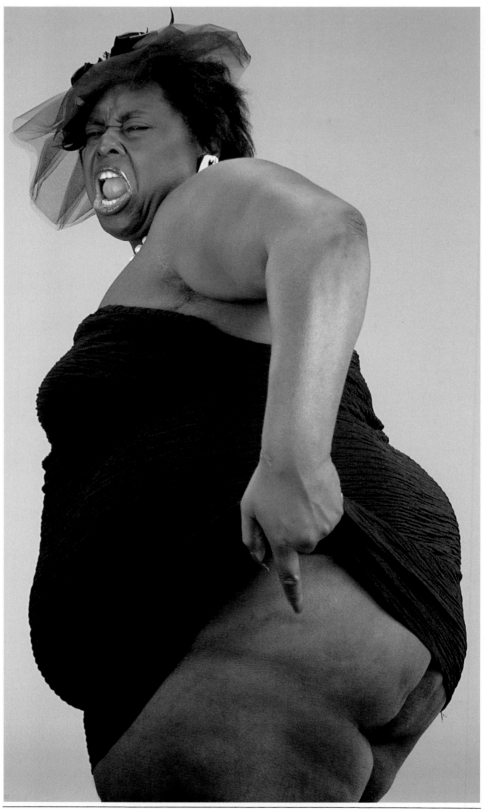

"One size fits all." All what?

□ HIPS & TIPS

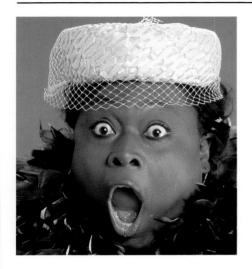

Alright, let's face more facts. There are a few drawbacks, to say the least, to being a Sister of Plenty. One of the drawbacks is that we're special, and when some people were making some things they didn't really think about us. I won't even dignify the absurd "One Size Fits All" notion by commenting on it. No, let's talk about more serious things. Theater seats in new malls; flying coach on any airline; wicker chairs; small plastic or wood folding chairs; small booths; these are just a few of of the natural hazards that Sisters of Plenty face in their everyday dealings. But what about the other hazards?

What other hazards? You know, the places we Sisters of Plenty have avoided like the plague. Such as the beach, honey, fat girls avoid the beach like married men avoid hickies. Pools—most of us would have to be held at gun point to go to a public pool. And the saddest and silliest of them all— smorgasbords. I've seen many a Sister of Plenty walking by a smorgasbord with lust in her eyes, dying to bust up inside, park her hams at a table and commit edacity and crapulence (that's a nice way of saying pig out, for you illiterates out there, kinda like poot is a nice way of saying fart). But does she dare approach the smorgasbord . . . no! And why? Because fat people aren't supposed to be seen eating in public. I don't know why, everybody knows we eat.

So when you have that little vacation. Where do you go? Well, first of all if you're gonna fly, go first class, or you'll find the friendly skies gripping at your hips tighter than you've been gripped by anything in the last fifteen years. For a Sister of Plenty to try and fly coach she either has to have one of two things: the courage of two cannibals having oral sex, or the IQ of a mung bean. And usually it's the latter. Let's face it, the airlines forgot about those of us who can't put our excess baggage in the overhead compartment. (Well, maybe some of us could, but Flo, how kinky would that be?)

As much as the whitewashed little cottage with the picket fence and the red brick walk, a two week vacation is part of the American Dream. So, let's get on with vacation tips for the heavy-hipped womanthang.

If you have beach phobia, the Islands aren't necessarily out. There are other things to do on the islands besides hang out on the white sand beaches, and bask in the warm tropical sun and splash about in the crystal clear refreshing blue water. You can always go to the mall. Everybody has a mall.

Or you could go to a Luau. Those island luaus are doozies sometimes. (Just be leery if they ask you to come naked with an apple in your mouth.)

Not to mention, there are always those northern islands, like the Aleutians, Iceland, Greenland and those islands off the coast of the North Pole. And as long as you're considering the Aleutians, you might as well give Alaska some thought. Did you know that men outnumber women seven to one in Alaska? Yes, Alaska's that kind of country where men are men and women are grateful. So what if you have to put on some snow-shoes and jump on a dog sled with a backpack full of dried whale blubber to get them. Nobody said that this life was going to be easy . . . especially the vacation part of it.

Personally, I like to vacation at a nice little all-you-can-eat sushi bar. Honey, I park my big legs up at that sushi bar and eat fish like Flipper, or Orca if you want to be technical.

I went to an all-you-can-eat sushi bar with Macho Puff, you know, man of my dreams Macho Puff, who abandoned me while I was writing my last book and proposed marriage to another woman while I was writing this one (oh well, a career girl's life is not pretty, and it's not easy). Anyway, Macho Puff and I went to an all-you-can-eat sushi bar. Unfortunately, they had a time limit on the all-you-can-eat special. It was only two hours. Well, after one hour and fifty minutes of serious sushi eating, Macho Puff orders twenty orders of Abalone, ten orders of yellowtail, fifteen orders of unagi, and a dozen California rolls.

Honey, that little tight-eyed sushi chef had the nerve to throw down his sushi knife and refuse to make it. He said we had eaten more sushi than the entire restaurant combined. Yes! Child, he told me that I ate an entire yellowtail by myself. You know that little short sucker had the nerve to tell moi, that the last time he saw anything like my eating was when they had catered the Sumo Wrestling Championships. Then he asked me if I was a Sumo wrestler! Well, Macho Puff got him straight. He told that little rickshaw jockey that if it truly was an all-you-can-eat sushi place, they would just put out buckets of fish and buckets of rice and piles of nouri sea weed wrap and let the people make their own.

Then his wife came out, looking like the Ho Chi Minh trail, spurting off in some obscure Asian dialect, (Japanese) and said that we were creating a disturbance and would have to leave the restaurant and should never come back.

I grabbed the heifer, and threatened to unslant those eyes, cause I'm a Detroit girl and we are not shy, honey. She said she knew karate and was not afraid of me. I told her I didn't care if she knew Chairman Mao, I'd tear that place up in there.

We got to tussling in that place. It got ugly. She tried ju-jitsu on me. It didn't work. She jumped back and said Hiya! and grabbed me by the arm. I twirled that heifer like she was a baton. When I got done beating butt as the Rams would say, there was rice paper, chopsticks, fortune cookies, and raw fish everywhere.

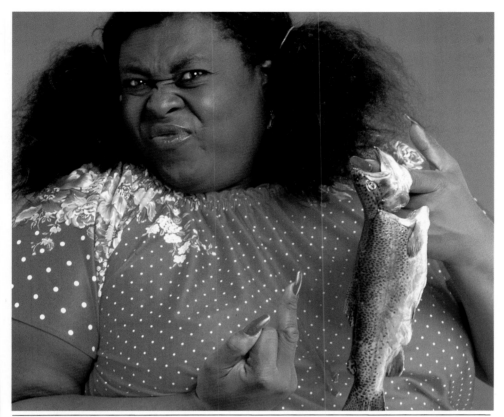

I don't care what they call it, think twice before putting anything raw and slimy in your mouth.

As I left I heard somebody speaking with a deep southern accent, I turned to see this Texan take his Wasabe, plop it in his mouth and turn to his wife and say, "ooouuuwee Ethyl...this is the hottest Guacomole!" ∎

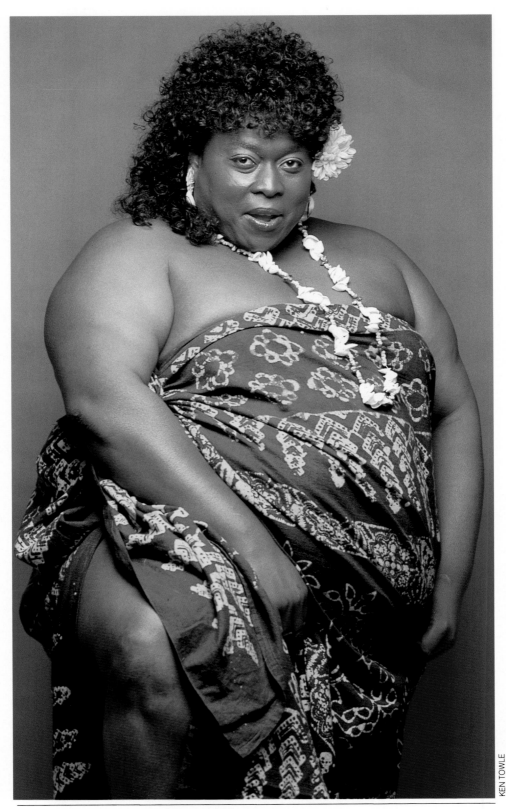

KEN TOWLE

If all else fails, slap on a sheet and call it a sarong.

☐ CAMOUFLAGING THE BULK

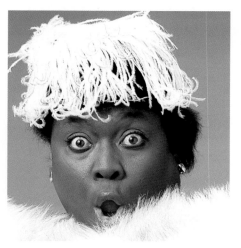

Alright, even though I've insisted for this entire book that the best defense is offense, and that you should be what you are and be proud or diet rationally and safely and change yourself, let's face it, some of you are going to do neither. And far be it from *moi*, to pass judgment. I didn't even pass judgement the last time I was in the confessional and a drunk priest opened the window and said, "Is there any paper on your side?" So why would I pass judgment if you decide that you want to be fat but look thin.

Okay, so let's get down to it. How then to hide the buns of Navarone? I know exactly what you're going through. I went through it myself. People are calling your panties thunder alley and clerks in offices are returning forms and saying "Excuse me, ma'am, but you put your zip code in the space where your weight is supposed to go." Yes I know.

Now, I won't mention any names, but certain high fashion models when they start pushing thirty the wrong way (in both waist and age) break out the basic blacks, the blazers and the big beads. When you see that, you know that muumuu season is right around the corner.

All of your reknowned designers say that simple, large straight, loose garments hide the excesses. Seeing that I don't believe in excess (there's never too much, there's just not enough being used) it's hard for me to think along those lines.

The other obvious way of camouflaging bulk, as they would say, is to use restraining devices. (No, I don't mean cuffs and shackles.) Girdles. Ever since woman put down the loin cloth she has been lacing corsets, tying trusses, squeezing into teddies and snapping girdles. The only problem with a girdle is if you're holding in some serious abundance, when you get your man home, it's kinda embarrassing when you take off your girdle and your feet disappear.

But then again, most of those fiends only want one thing and they don't care what they have do to get it, even if that means rolling you in flour and going for the wet spot.

However, I say the best way to disguise abundance is to creatively place it. For example, don't pull your stomach in, push it up for added cleavage. A girl can never have too much tit.

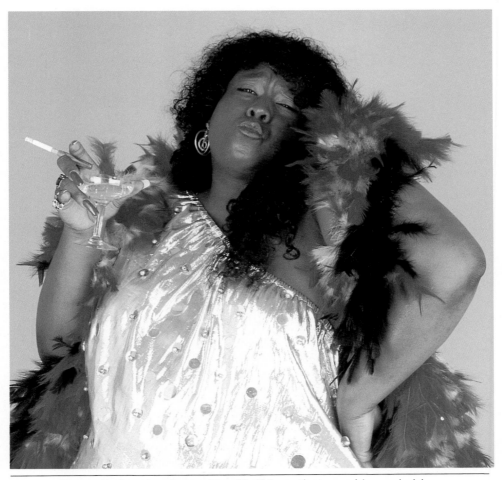

Cover those strech marks with things that sparkle and shine.

Ruffles and layers. Honey, break out the ruffled skirts and the gypsy bangles and give them layer upon layer of party dress. They will just automatically assume that you're not that big. Although, let's face it honey, you'll never fool a flight of stairs or a wicker chair.

The other way to camouflage bulk is to do as the cobra does: blind your victims. It's kinda like, well, if I may quote myself, "Los Angeles is like a rich old spinster, she covers her wrinkles with things that sparkle and shine and are certain to catch any young man's eye." And that's the t, honey. Give them so much diamond, ruby and sapphire that they don't notice anything else. I promise you, if you put enough diamonds around your neck, they will never notice the four chins hanging above them. Ruby ankle bracelets unfortunately aren't as effective with fat ankles however. ■

☐ WORKOUT BLUES

Well the peace rally is over, and the hippies all are dead
People aren't talking politics, they're talking aerobics instead.
So I've traded in my girdle for a pair of running shoes,
Cause I'm the 70s emerging woman, singing the 80s workout blues!

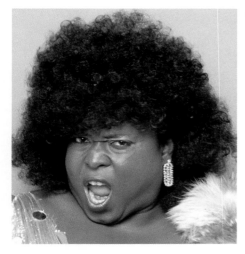

Yes it's true, honey, it's a brand new day. Girls are running for that gym like they're giving something away. Everybody is swearing that they'll have muscles in their eyelashes and ripples in their nose. People are driven. Just last week a woman died at the gym screaming, "Give me red meat!"

People have gone even further than that. Child, the other day a bunch of hussies busted into Burger King and said, "hold the burgers just give us the lettuce, honey, those special orders do upset us!" Is nothing sacred?

The sale of sprouts and designer sweats is at an all time high. Skinny heifers, with no hips at all are walking around with their heads in the sky. Women that in the good old days would have been laid up in a county hospital on an I.V. filled with vegetable oil are now claiming to be sex symbols. Although I still haven't heard anyone of them commit to either sex ... and I suppose I could say something, but people who live in glass slums shouldn't throw trash. But you know they do, so let's get on with it.

Exercise! It's a neurotic obsession, honey. Maybe these white women, who spend their days doing absolutely nothing but sitting up in a tennis outfit, eating celery, buried in peanut butter and wheat thins by the bushel, watching one soap opera after another, need to exercise. But us women of more color, and less capital, do not need to exercise.

Now think about it. You get up in the morning and you make your old man something to eat. (And if you ain't got an old man, that's even worse, because you've tossed and turned all night, so you've definitely burned off some calories). Anyway, back to the typical day of a woman of greater color and lesser capital; after you make your old man's breakfast, you push him out the door. Then you do the dishes, clean the house, take a shower, throw on your face. Now that's a good 5,000 calories burned off right there.

Not to mention as the day wears on, your auxilliary husband is bound to come over for a little tit and tat, so to speak. So that's another 3,000 calories burned. And on any given day a utility man, or some random bill collector is bound to show up at your door; needless to say you won't have the money so you'll have to think of more creative ways to get that bill taken care of. Another 2,500 calories down the old schmazoo.

By this time your auxillary husband's wife is calling up on the phone saying she found your panties in her old man's pocket and she wants you to keep your hands off. To which, of course, you have to explain (in a polite but firm fashion) that if that man was really her old man, he would've told you so this morning when he was leaving your boudoir.

And when you think about it, it's the practical exercise that's going to be our salvation. Expecting a Sister of Plenty to get into running out to the gym and spending her days exercising in public, deep in the heart of Weight Nazi territory is like waiting for Diana Ross to go back to the Supremes. It ain't likely to happen; not in this life, anyway. Besides, there must be life after sit-ups . . .

And all of the exercises that people do at the gym are so painful, not to mention dangerous! Have you ever thought about what would happen if too many Sisters of Plenty bent over to touch their toes at the same time? Can you imagine, especially here in earthquake-sensitive California? It could be disasterous. Think about it on an international level. Imagine . . . If all the Sisters of Plenty in the world bent over to touch their toes at the same time, it could throw the earth off its axis and out of its orbit and we could end up hurling through space endlessly. Do you know what that would do to our economy . . .

Not to mention astro-physiological-psychosomatic-inter-universal space entwinement. (For those of you who aren't from California, that means that Jewish boys would start playing professional football and basketball, W.A.S.P.s would suddenly find themselves well-endowed and inclined to prefer music with a beat. Negroes would start becoming doctors, lawyers and accountants by the thousands, homosexuals would become untidy, and lesbians would start bathing regularly and stop drinking beer.) Scary thought, isn't it?

If that's not enough calories burned off for you, then I have included some civilized day to day exercises that you can do in the privacy and comfort (or discomfort) of your own home.

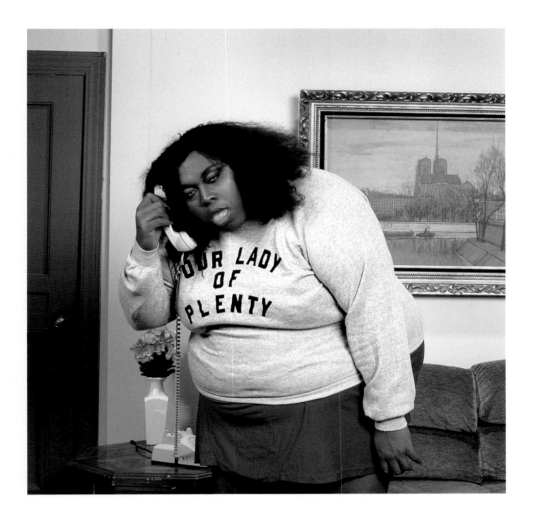

■ The Phone Dash

The phone dash is a simple but effective exercise. What you do is, wait for the phone to ring.

Now, if you have no friends and your phone seldom rings, then do this: Go out and bounce a bunch of checks and give them your correct phone number. Your phone will ring ... constantly.

Now back to the phone dash. What you do is you wait for the phone to ring. When the phone rings you ask the party calling if they will hold on while you change phones. You hang up the phone and try to make it to your second phone before the line disconnects.

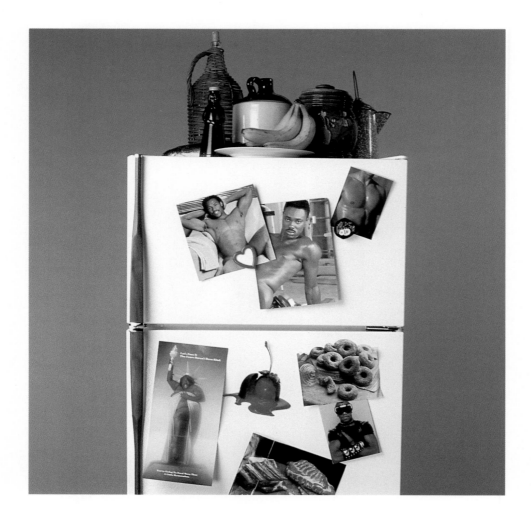

■ Refrigerator Curls

What one appliance, besides the microwave, do we use most? That's right—the refrigerator. So this is a very simple exercise and you don't have to go out of your way to do it. All you do is remember that each time you go to the refrigerator, instead of opening the door once, you open it ten times, then you get what you want.

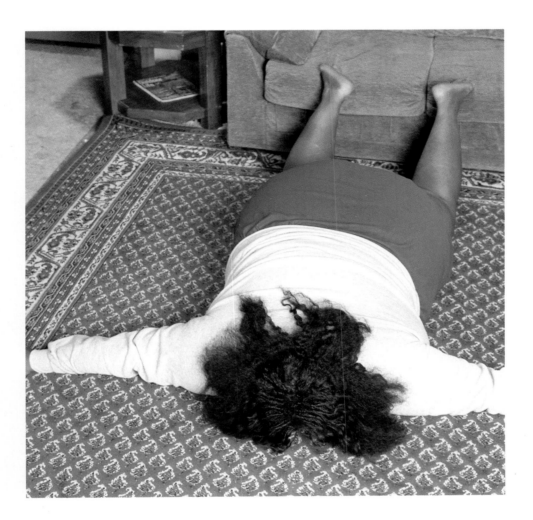

■ Splats

Doing a 'Splat' seems simple at first. All you have to do is get down on your knees. And God knows, you've done that once or twice (to pray, I mean). It's after you're on your knees that the hard part comes. Right, wishful thinking. Anyway, you allow yourself to fall, stomach first, on the floor. Your body should make a loud "SPLAT" sound. That's why they're called 'Splats', Mary Beth!

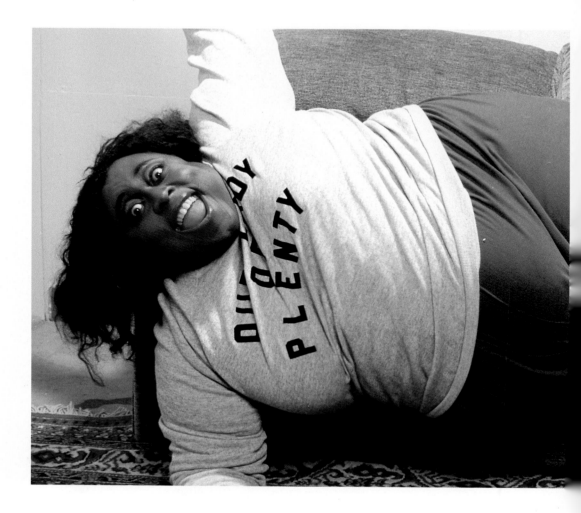

■ Sofa Twists

This exercise is just like a good Irish girl—sweet and simple. All you do is lay on the sofa, and once every five minutes turn onto your opposite side. If you're really energetic, then you can do it once every three minutes. If you're totally jocked out, do it once every minute. If you're on drugs do it every fifteen seconds.

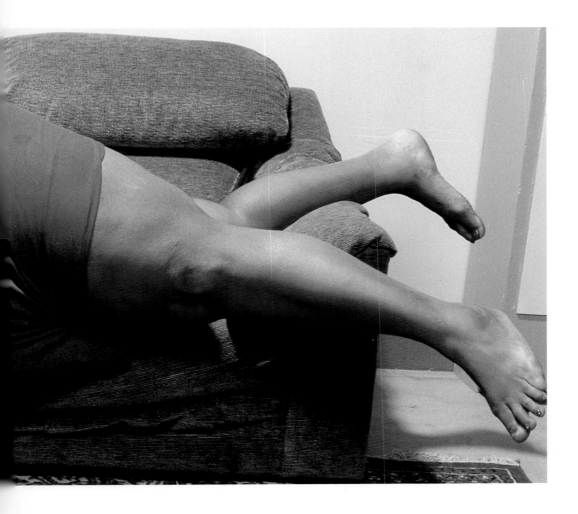

■ Bathercise

Besides being a lot of fun, this is one exercise that will leave you clean instead of sweaty when you're done. Run yourself a big bubble bath. Then take some dish soap, (I recommend Palmolive) and squirt it all over your buttois, until your rear is nice and slippery. Get in the bathtub and turn on some music. Do not let the radio get too close to the bath tub. A radio in a bathtub is some ugly t.

Anyway, turn on a jazz station, and slide around to the music in the bathtub. You'll find it most invigorating.

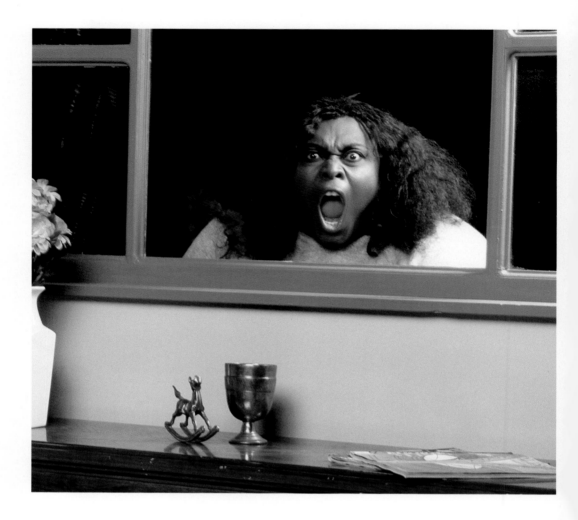

■ Peek-Ups

Like I say in the opening, this is an exercise for voyeurs only. What you do is, you go to the window where you watch your neighbor. Squat down so that your head is below the window sill, then you pop up periodically, trying to, of course, catch some dirt going on. This is great for trimming the thighs, and I even know a woman who got rid of a double chin by doing this exercise. (Of course it was shot off by an irate neighbor ... but she lost it just the same.)

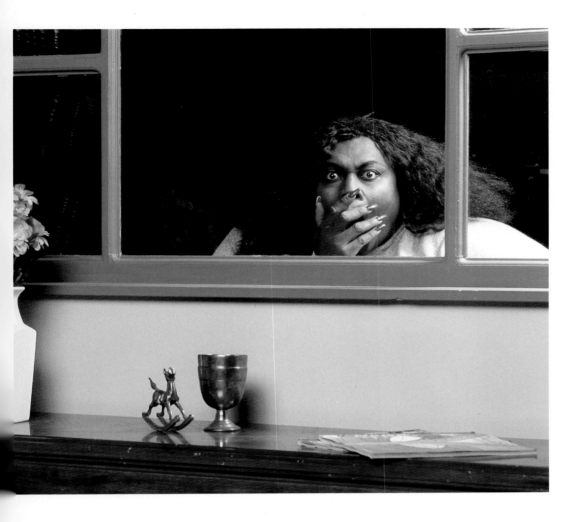

■ Buffalo Wallow Woman Routine

T his exercise is a lot of fun, to say the least. It's also very easy to do. All you do is go outside to a park, or on your lawn, and imagine that you are a huge buffalo, and that you are very warm and itchy. Then you get down on the ground and roll around for an hour or so.

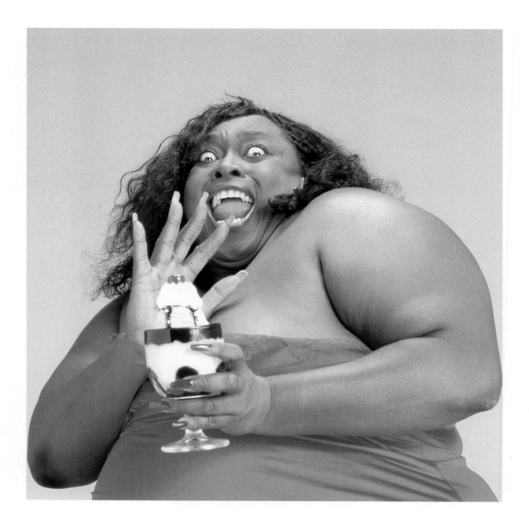

■ Food Hunt

Sometimes in this life we have to look to others who don't have our problem as a source of ideas as to how to handle our problem. Well, I decided, who spent years on television in a bathing suit? That's right, Lloyd Bridges. And why was he so lean and trim? Because of all the exercise that he got on *Sea Hunt*. I have consequently developed an exercise that even you inland girls can do that is comparable to *Sea Hunt* for us Sisters of Plenty . . . that's right . . . Food Hunt.

It's a very simple exercise, all you do is get a friend or a semi-enemy to hide all of your food around the house. Then whenever you get hungry you'll have to make a mad dash to find it before it spoils . . . just like Lloyd had to find the bomb before it blew up the cruise ship. (And believe me honey, you'll be searching harder for that Haagen Daz than Lloyd ever did for any bomb.)

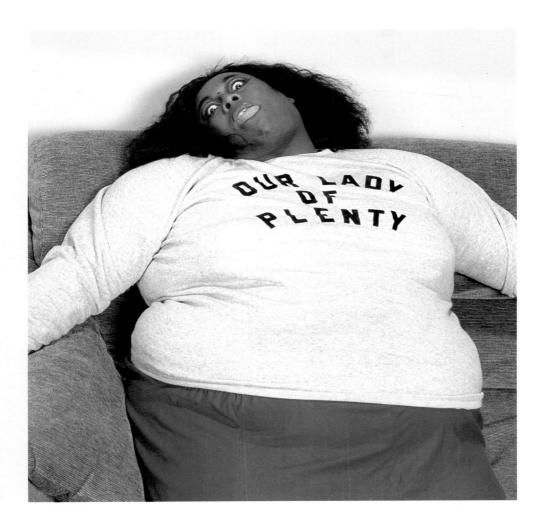

■ Sludge Downs

Find yourself a very sturdy chair, and plop down in it and exhale. Do this at least twelve times a day.

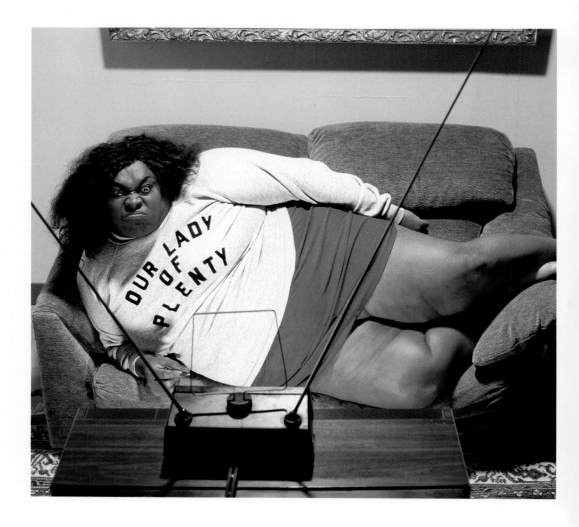

■ Soap Opera Ups

This little exercise is simpler yet. All you have to do is get yourself a reclining chair and get in front of the television. If you don't have a reclining chair, use your couch; just lay on your side. Now turn on your favorite soap opera, and every time something illegal, immoral or sexual happens, just lift your head. That'll tighten those neck muscles, honey.

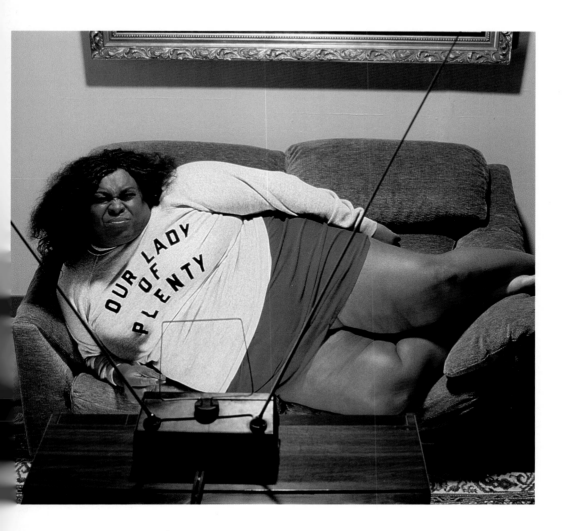

■ Channel Touches

This is a simple yet practical exercise that is suited to the lifestyle of every Sister of Plenty. The only equipment that you need is a remote channel changer and a television. Now what you do is you take the channel changer and you place it out of your immediate grasp, then every commercial break you stretch to the channel changer and get it and flip through the channels and then put it back out of your immediate grasp.

If you want to do some extreme exercise, change the channel manually at the commercial break by getting up and walking to the television.

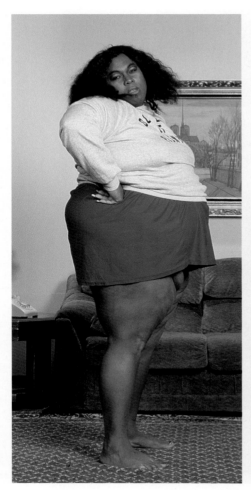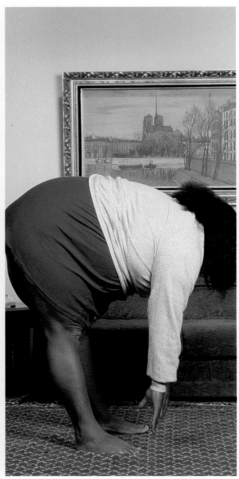

■ Heaves

This exercise is kind of like the time a man came up to me and said, "Excuse me darling, but are you a navajo?" I said, "no." The man replied, "Well then what kind of 'ho' are you?" It's all in a look. Some students of kinesiology and exercise might call this exercise "Toe Touches," but you and I know that a Sister of Plenty does not touch her toes, not in peace time, anyway.

Granted this may look like your touching your toes, and you may even touch them, but remember that's neither here nor there. What you do is this. You pretend that you're dreadfully hung-over and you're about to blow chunks. You bend over like you're about to pray to the porcelain god, and the weight of your wombacious breasts should take you straight on down to the floor. Now here comes the exercise. Try to straighten back up.

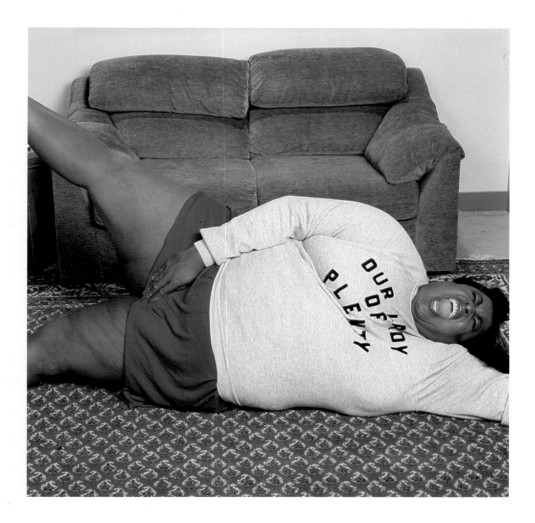

■ Medullah Cuspettes

The medullah cuspette is perhaps a painful exercise, but the rewards are many. Besides, exercise is kinda like love in that way, "It ain't no good, until it hurts a little bit." (And if the truth be told, it ain't really no good until it hurts a lot.) Well it's too early in the morning for me to jump up and go to testifying on such a serious subject—so back to the cuspettes.

You lay on your side and you raise your thigh in the air in a scissor-kick fashion until you can feel the remnants of your bridal trousseau tugging at your hope chest so to speak. The rest of your body will fall into a natural fit of contortion. Do that as many times as you can and in no time you'll be over this exercise.

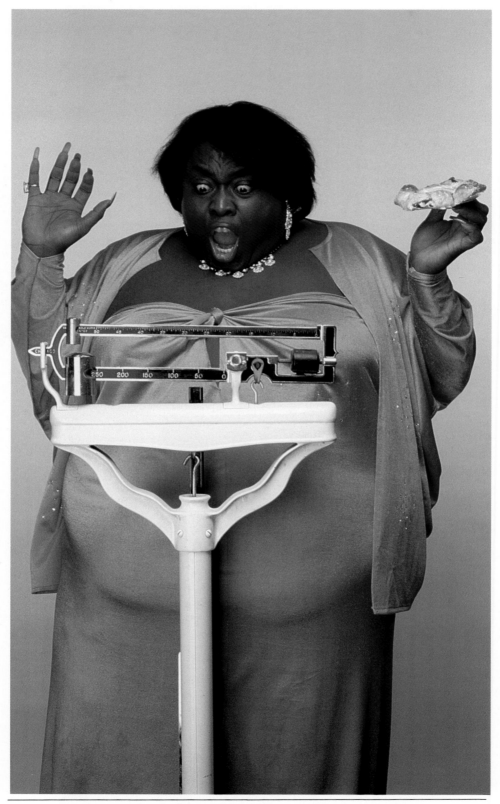

Read it and weep. And if you can't read it, weep anyway.

☐ CALORIES

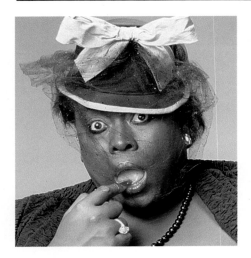

For two days now, I've been walking around here with a long face, lookin' like a piece of chewed string, avoiding this essay like it had tentacles and secreted puss. Why? I don't know. I guess it's just something from way back when Sisters of Plenty and calories were always just mortal enemies. Well, the fact of the matter is that calories are not really our enemies.

So what exactly is a calorie? Technically a calorie is the amount of heat required at a pressure of one atmosphere to raise the temperature of one gram of water one degree Celsius (centigrade). So what the hell does that mean? You got me. I have absolutely no idea. So don't ask me what it has to do with the price of mumu's at Lane Bryant's. It sounds totally harmless if you ask me. What's a gram of water? And what's one little old degree on the scale? Nothing, right? Well, we all know that when you start piling those calories on top of each other, one after the other, like Sandy Duncan eating Wheat Thins, you've got trouble.

Calories are our friends. I know, how could I have the unmitigated gall, the uncurtailed temerity, the unbridled audacity, to claim that calories are our friends? Calories—the reason we're at the mercy of such clothiers as "The Forgotten Woman", "House of Plenty", "More to Love", Lane Bryant", and "Omar's." Calories—the reason you spent four days in the hospital last summer 'cause your husband was making love to you and in the heat of it your stomach fell back over your face and you almost suffocated. Calories—the reason you break out in hives when you see patio furniture. Calories—the reason you have to put erase on your neck.

Au contraire, mon ami! Calories are really our only hope, if we want to get thin. You see you have to have a guide to go by. And I know, it's heartbreaking when you find out that fried chicken has 568 calories in it and that sprouts have 45. It's terrible news. All the good things have a lot of calories in them. But just remember this, 10,000 calories, a Sister of Plenty does not make. That's right. Even if you totally oink out in a day and have 15,000 calories, if you come back to your normal maintenance requirement of calories you'll be all right. So fear not.

Being afraid of calories is like having been afraid of doing the "dirty deed" when you were in high school. Once you lost your virginity you were fine. The fear went away, and you started to learn about other things that you

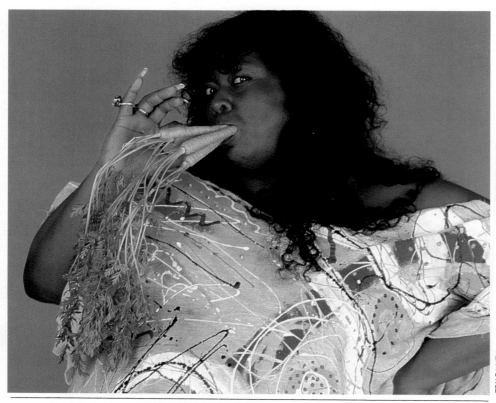

KEN TOWLE

Carrots are not a girl's best friend.

needed to suit your new lifestyle, such as diaphrams, control-top pantyhose and make-up. The same is true with calories. Once you jump in there and start counting those calories on a daily basis it won't be so bad. You'll learn that you can mix and match. When you're having the heavy duty caloric meats, then you throw in the light weight vegetables. It will be a piece of cake. Ooops, did I say that? Perish the thought!

The final thing to remember about counting calories, and this calorie guide in particular, is that the calories found here are approximates. There is no need to get neurotic about counting calories. Trust me, your body is not going to explode over a 100 calorie discrepancy. Don't punish yourself, that is the key. If you punish yourself and try to eat rabbit food you're gonna fail, because you're not a rabbit, Blanche! ■

☐ WAYS TO BURN OFF CALORIES (Creatively)

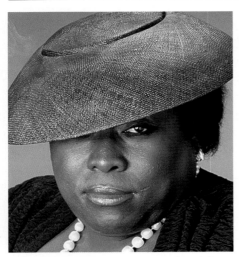

Everybody knows if you go down to the gym and you aerobicize for hours, work out on the weight machines, and jog up this hill and down that hill you're bound to trim off some pounds. But honey ... how boring ... how drab ... how lesbian-like!

Now, let's talk about truth. Do we not get up in the morning and go to work all day long and half the night, too, with one little lunch break, a coffee break here and there, and maybe a short pee in the late afternoon? Do we not do this to make our lives more pleasant and ourselves happier? Right? Am I speaking truth, Sisters of Plenty? Indeed, indeed! Now, why should we take our good hard earned money and give it to some skinny heifer, who we don't know, and even if we did, probably wouldn't like, to join her gym? For what? To sit up in a room full of fat floozies, flouncing, and flopping around, like a school of dying marlin, listening to some tired top-forty tune that has driven you crazy on the way to and from work for months now. Honey, please! It just ain't normal. I can't believe that fully grown women can't find something better to do, or at least something more fun to do, than look at their neighbors' saggy behind bouncing to the beat of *Private Dancer* for hours. Tell the truth, wouldn't you rather be sitting up in a cocktail lounge gripping onto the latest festive tropical libation, giving some lonely soldier heavy eyelash, much winkage and serious attitude? Even the old rerun sitcoms on the independent TV stations are better than jogging.

Who really likes to jog? Maybe five people, ten at most, who were traumatized in the birth canal, and have tendon and ligiment fetishes. I'll be the first one to say it. If you see me jogging, it means two things ... 1. somebody is after me, and 2. I can't find my switchblade.

It's a communist plot. That's right, those big, ugly, manly-lookin' Russian heifers from the Olympic shot put, tractor pulling and javelin catching teams, are trying to take our men. Umhhmm, that's the t, honey. They own these gyms, and when we get done aerobicizing, honey, there ain't gonna be nothing feminine, soft, and desirable left. Where there once were scenic curves there'll be nothing but straight turnpike all the way. And honey, it's gonna be the highway to heartache.

There are better ways to exercise. I mean there just has got to be doesn't there? Of course there is. And I am the one to tell you how to burn off calories in a creative and fun fashion.

ACTIVITY	NUMBER OF CALORIES USED
Putting On Your Face:	
If you're a Purina Model	1,275
If you're a "1"	1,000
If you're a "5"	850
If you're a "10"	500
If you're *really* a "10"	0
Mild flirting	25
Moderate flirting	50
Serious flirting	75
This is *The Man* flirting	125
This is *The Man* and he's getting away flirting	1,000
Homewrecking:	
A marriage on the rocks	500
A weak marriage	750
A good marriage with a weak man	1,250
A good marriage with a good man	4,000
A good marriage with a good woman	40,000
Giving Birth To The Blues:	
An easy birth	1,000
A somewhat difficult birth	2,000
A hard birth	4,000
Triplets	10,000
Disco-ing:	
Going through the motions	50
Hard and heavy	1,000
Diva disco-ing	2,000
Decorating:	
Normal Suburban	400
Massive Renovation	1,000
Gay Baroque	25,000

What I have decided to do is list a few daily activities that one might partake of and suggest, figuratively, and approximately speaking, how many calories a girl might burn off partaking of these daily activities. ■

ACTIVITY	NUMBER OF CALORIES USED
Shopping:	
For the necessities	50
Light shopping	100
Moderate shopping	550
Heavy shopping	1,000
JAP shopping	12,579
Bead Reading:	
Gentle rebuke	0
Harsh Words	50
Serious verbal conflict	75
Cat fight	100
Drag Queen reading	1,000
Tussling:	
Light scuffle	100
Brief fight	250
Brawl	500
Knock down drag 'em out	1,000
Showdown over a man between 2 Italian girls	25,000
Showdown over a man between 2 black girls	50,000
Showdown over a man between 2 WASP girls	0
Doing The Dirty Deed:	
Terrible deed	0
Bad deed	50
Average deed	500
Good deed	850
Great deed	1,950
Make me write bad checks deed	5,678

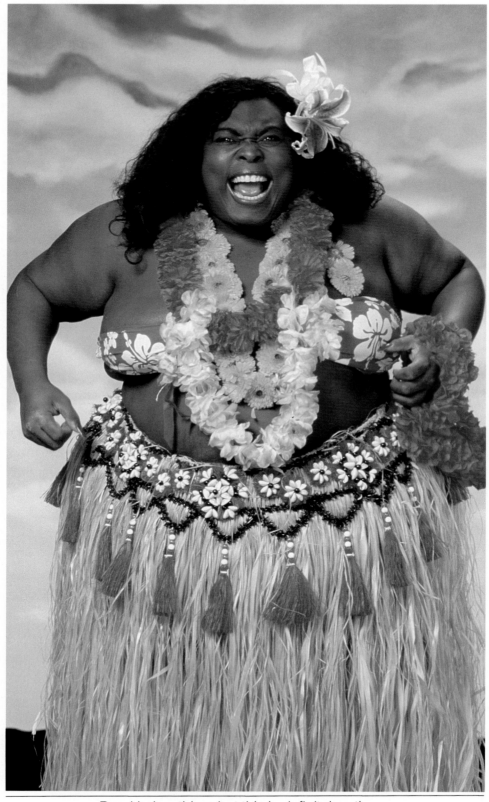

Don Ho is a thing, but this is definitely a thang.

☐ THINGS & THANGS

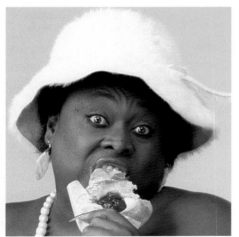

Sometimes trying to make people understand my simple command of the English language is like taking Stevie Wonder to a Marcel Marceau recital. A prime example is the difference between a "thing" and a "thang". I tried to clarify that difference in my last book, (*You've Had Worse Things In Your Mouth*), but for those of you who ain't well read, I will give you a brief definition.

Toledo, Ohio is a thing; Hollywood is a thang. Queen Elizabeth is a thing; B.B. King is a thang. The Moral Majority is a thing; The rest of us are thangs. A London Fog Raincoat is a thing; A floor-length fox fur is a thang. A Dodge Dart is a thing; A Maserati is a thang. Zsa Zsa Gabor is a thing; Susan Anton is a thang. Jane Fonda is a thing; I am a thang.

Okay, enough. Anyway, I have chosen to call this next section *Things & Thangs* for just this reason, because I have included a great many items which go into our mouths, some of which are things, and some of which are thangs. (Unfortunately there never seems to be enough thangs, if you know what I mean.) Anyhow, I have tried to give you a relatively accurate and somewhat comprehensive guide for the woman of the eighties.

I found I needed to divide this section into two separate sections, *Musts* and *Maybes*. Now, everybody knows I'm as liberal as a Jew with a flat tire in a black neighborhood, so far be it from moi, to pass judgement on which foods are *Musts* and which foods are *Maybes*; after all, I don't have any shakey commodity investments lying around, and God knows the only stock I own is soup stock—and I don't mean forty shares of Campbell's either. So I will give you as clear and as unadulterated an opinion as you're gonna get.

However, fate has her wenchly ways, and I have to divide these things on some basis. So I have decided to do so on the basis of which things in my past seem to be Musts, and which things seem to be Maybes. Which brings me to a little story. Don't you just love my little stories? Oh yeah? Well then you shouldn't have bought this book!

My girlfriend, Kitacious, was marrying this airplane pilot that she had picked up, ooops, I mean met in Anchorage. The marriage was supposed to be the following day, in Vegas, during his two-hour layover on his flight from Anchorage to Cleveland. Well, the other girls and I decided that such a traditional wedding deserved an equally traditional shower.

We decided to hold the girl's shower at Chez Moi, on Lady's Night. (I know, what does all this have to do with Musts and Maybe's . . . just hold on to your panties, I'm getting there, sugar.) Well, before we held her shower, we went out for a pre-shower meal at the Golden Bull (the girl's favorite restaurant). Well, I happen to have had a few slices of pie. That night I was wearing my red fishtail dress and black fishnet stockings with the rhinestone seam up the back . . . your basic shower wear. I had on a pair of black panties, with a rhinestone broach in the front, (just in case you slip and fall and your dress flies over your head, I think it's always good to have something down there that will catch a little light.

Well, we weren't in Chez Moi more than ten minutes before the elastic in my panties gave way. Honey, my drawers hit the floor. So, I did the only thing that a sterling example of feminine decorum would do, I stepped out of them, and gave them a gentle drop-kick into a nearby potted palm. I had every intention of getting them at last call. Needless to say, better intentions than mine have fallen by the wayside. In my drunken stupor, ooops, I mean, in my slight inebriation—I forgot and left my lingerie in the potted palm.

Well, the next day, much to my chagrin, the manager of Chez Moi called me up and said, "Look, honey, we found some drawers in one of our palms that could only belong to you."

Horrified and humiliated, I began to apologize, only to have the manager say, "Oh, don't apologize, we were calling to ask you if we could rent these panties from you because they're killing the aphids and mites in our plants in a cold-blooded fashion."

As much as I'm into public service—and you know I've tried hard to serve the public, I must admit, I was a bit taken aback by the thought of a cocktail lounge using my panties for pest control. But I did give my consent.

So, what does this have to do with Musts and Maybes? It was that pie! If I hadn't eaten that pie my panties would never have exploded at Chez Moi and ended up in the potted palms. That's why I have decided to put Pie at the top of the Maybe list. And you know what they say, "Five minutes on the lips and five years on the hips." So I've examined my hips as well. All the foods that I've found on my hips I have put on the Maybe list and the rest are on the Must. ∎

□ MUSTS

There are only two "Musts" in this world: Death and Taxes. However, here are a few other things and thangs that come close.

■ MEAT

So what if the only way you could ever see your toes is via satellite? Big deal if you work part time selling shade space at parades. It has nothing to do with red meat directly. Indirectly, granted, those five whoppers, two whopper juniors, four orders of fries and case of Tab from your last visit to Burger King may very well indeed be on your thighs. But let us look at the facts; it's not the red meat that we eat, but the quantity of red meat. Now, I know that a lot of these skinny little granola & sprout heifers are swearing that red meat causes everything from cellulite to unemployment. Lies. The fact of the matter is, red meat is a good source of protein, though it be higher in fat content than chicken or fish. And it does tend to be more difficult to digest. But there is something to be said for instincts in this life, and people didn't start eating beef because Jupiter was in retrograde with Mars. Human beings are carnivrous, and if you don't believe me, just take the Greyhound to Detroit and get off the bus.

I will agree that for the most part we do eat more red meat than we need to. We also pay more taxes than we should but what's a girl to do? The truth is the light, and there is no certain amount of red meat that one should or should not eat. The key to being successful in the final diet is learning to listen to your instincts, and if your honest instincts tell you to eat five legs of lamb, a case of pork chops and a light beer, then go for it. Of course, the other trick is determining when your instincts are talking and when your neuroses are flapping their proverbial gums. Heavy, huh? Well I'm a heavy womanthang.

■ BREAD

One of the first mistakes people make when they are dieting is that they don't eat bread. You'll end up looking like an old field in southern Mississippi if you don't eat your bread—and looking like anything in Mississippi is not good. As usual I have calculated it according to the single slice. Since most breads come sliced, this is a little more exact this time, as far as measures go.

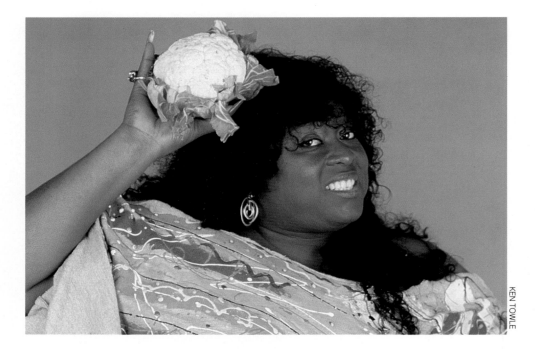

KEN TOWLE

■ VEGETABLES, LEGUMES & THANGS

Some of the great beauties of our times, like Zsa Zsa Gabor and Yuliis Ruval, maintain that vegetables make your skin glow. I'm sure this is probably true, and if anybody would know about that kind of thing those girls would. I'm also sure Estee Lauder and Clinique are none the poorer for it, as I'm sure those girls probably know something about that, too.

Of course, I am also revered in certain camps as one of the great beauties of our time. Now, I have found that it is true that fresh vegetables like carrots, lettuce and cucumber do something to enhance a girl's beauty. However, I find that french fries have had a great deal to do with my own special glow.

Speaking of that glow, and the responsibilities of being a great beauty, let me just say that it ain't easy, honey. Youth gather outside my boudoir window, to get a glimpse of my pulchritude in the dawn light. And sometimes that can be rough on a girl. Especially if you wake up looking like somebody threw your face on your head with a pitchfork, and all the lines you gave the men at the saloon the night before have come to rest around your eyes. That says nothing of the fact that your well kept coiffure is nappier than the southwest corner of a sheep's behind in the morning.

But, even though I was overlooked by the committee that selected California's ten most beautiful women, I manage not to let my fans down and the key to my success, again, I have to say, is french fries.

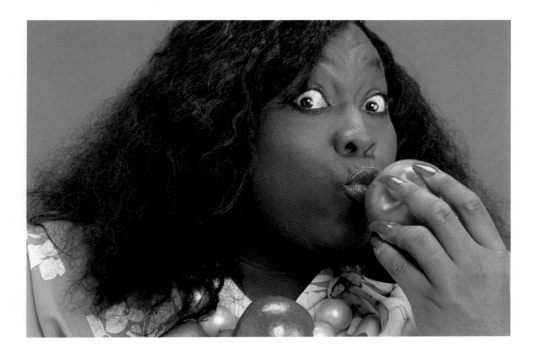

■ FRUIT

You're absolutely wrong. I'm not going to make any of the obvious comments you might think I would make. If anybody mentions your hairdresser, honey it will be you.

I'm going to talk about the professional things, since this is purely a professional endeavor. Well, anyway, let's talk about fruit.

Fruit is very good for you and it travels through your system like a gigolo through your checking account. As you will notice, some fruits are considerably higher in calories than other fruits. That depends on the sugar content. You know, it's kinda like us womanthangs—a couple of us might look alike, act alike, even live in the same neighborhood, but when you get down to some close investigation by a real discerning eye you learn that some of us are just sweeter than others. That's called sugar content.

For example, a bite of moi would be considerably higher in calories than a bite of say, Queen Elizabeth, though we're both Queens, and we both base a lot of our security in the reliability of the fleet, so to speak. It's just that I'm much higher in sugar content—especially brown sugar. You know that coarse, sweet, pungent, soft, unrefined sugar.

■ FISH

Now, most diets will have you eating so much fish that you'll be breathing through your cheeks. The fact of the matter is, that fish is an excellent source of protein, that it is low in calories and cholesterol, but then so is sperm, and I wouldn't recommend an overabundance of that either. However, I have to say I've never heard of a girl getting diamonds, trips or furs for eating fish. Never mind, forget I said that. Back to the issue at hand. Fish. If you like fish, go for it, it's a great source of protein and it's very low in calories and real good for you. If you don't like fish, then just get on up the street. Don't eat it. Although I will say this, there are lots of different types of fish, like there's lots of different types of men, and when I hear a person say they don't like fish, I tend to think they have only tried a couple of types a couple of ways. Try lots of different types of fish, lots of different ways. However, when I hear people say they don't like men, I tend to think I'm in the wrong bar.

■ POULTRY

The only thing I have to say about chicken is that I know a few people that are serving time over them. As far as turkeys go, I could do a thesis on turkeys, the do's and don'ts. Instead I'll just give you the calories and let you continue on in your quest to not look like your stretch pants were put on with a spray gun.

■ YOGURT

Asking me to talk about yogurt is like asking Diana Ross to talk about marrying poor men. I just don't know a thing about it. You see, black folks don't eat yogurt. Well, I'm sure that somewhere there's some Oreo sitting up in a cafeteria in a pair of topsiders and a LaCoste shirt, talking about snow skiing, eating yogurt. But he ain't here, so you're stuck with moi, and before I'd eat yogurt I'd walk through hell, carrying a backpack full of gasoline, wearing a straw teddie and rice paper pumps. (Do you think that was over stated?)

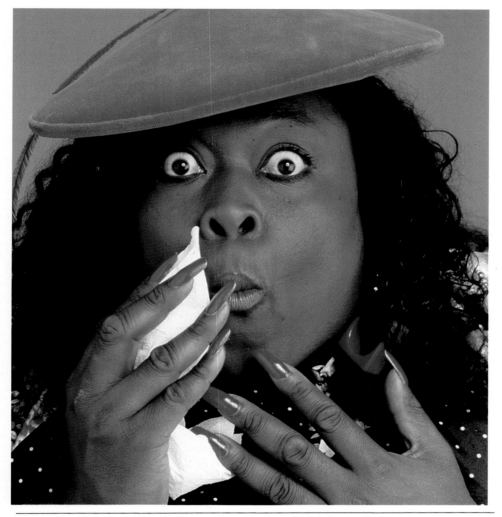

I'll take an order of pie—hold the guilt.

☐ **MAYBES**

Well as Janis said, "Maybe, maybe, maybe . . ." Of course she was talking about love, and then again . . . so am I. God knows, how many people do you know that have traded in their old man for a Big Mac and a large order of fries and a hot cherry pie? And in some cases rightfully so, cause a Big Mac, Fries and cherry pie has a lot more meat, grease and sweetness . . . not to mention that special sauce, than some of these men.

Anyway, here you will find the things that they claim that you don't absolutely need in this world. Of course, if my publisher would let me do this according to my philosophy I would put everything on this list, except one good man. Cause everybody knows that in this world all you really need is one good man . . . and even though it ain't much . . . honey, it's every little thang. (Using the term figuratively speaking . . . I hope.)

■ CAKE

One of my adversaries said that the men don't call me brown sugar because I'm sweet but because I'm so unrefined. Alright, I'll admit it, my family tree is a bush—and I'm not talking about George, honey. But what do you want from a girl who the doctor slapped on the butt & asked her to moo on the day she was born? And I know rumour has it that the only thing holding up my dress is a couple of low riding chins and a city ordinance. So where do I get off having the cheap untailored temerity to suggest that somebody eat cake on a diet? After all, surely I couldn't think that I was Marie Antoinette. (Although I don't know why not, since half the queens in Hollywood think they're Marilyn Monroe trapped in a totally buffed, salon-tanned, boy's body;) Anyway, it's true that sometimes when I go to the beach even the tugboats don't whistle. But then again, who was the Surf Queen of 1986? You guessed it—moi! And you know what my itsy bitsy, teeny weeny bikini was featuring—that's right, honey, cake. And as for the measurements for this section, I list the calories in one slice ... how big is a slice? Well dah'ling that depends on whose wielding the knife.

■ CANDY

Most people will tell you that candy is one of the last things you need on a diet. I say, the last thing you need is somebody gettin' up in your face, talkin' out of their neck about what you should and should not have. On my diet, the *last* diet, you can have anything you want, just as long as you count the calories. Now, granted there are a lot of calories in candy, but so what? Every now and then a girl just needs to eat a few Hershey bars. Hershey bars, Baby Ruth's, Butterfingers, Almond Joys, Mounds and Snickers, are some of the few dependable pleasures left on this earth.

Remember the key word in my diet is indulge. Indulge, indulge, indulge. Just don't over indulge and lose sight of your goal. Remember this is like daddy used to say, "One monkey don't stop no show." And that's the 't' too, honey. One little candy bar or two, or even if you've had all of your calories for the day and you eat six candy bars, your diet's not ruined. It's when you get all bent out of shape over eating the six candy bars and start feeling guilty and frustrated and like a failure that you give up and it's the surrender not the battle wounds that defeat a girl in a war against herself.

So remember, honey, you're not the United Nations, you're just an obscure Third World country full of turmoil and corruption and you're bound to have setbacks, so take them in stride and when they happen just throw your head back and act real white.

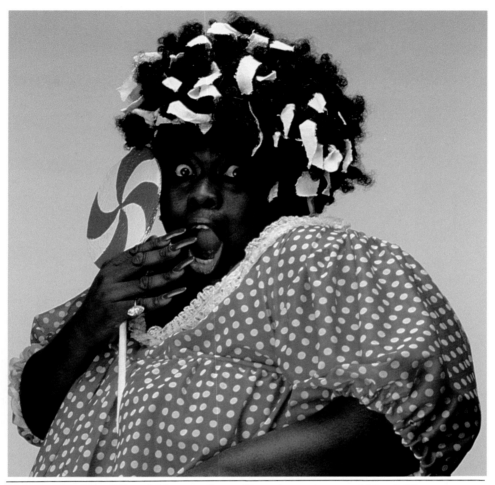

As a little girl I was often offered candy—and I took it!

■ PIES

Trying to zero in on what constitutes an exact slice of pie is like using a tortilla for a diaphram — it's an iffy situation at best. The only thing you can really do is just go for what you know and hope the gods are in a good mood and smiling on you. So when I say "one slice" I mean roughly a six oz. piece of pie, give or take an ounce or so.

■ COOKIES

Talking about cookies is like women talking about their husbands; it's all relative, 'cause what's a nut log to one girl might be a short bread to somebody else. So when I say one, I mean one typical-sized cookie. And we all know that even though there is no such thing as "average" or "normal", there is such a critter as "typical."

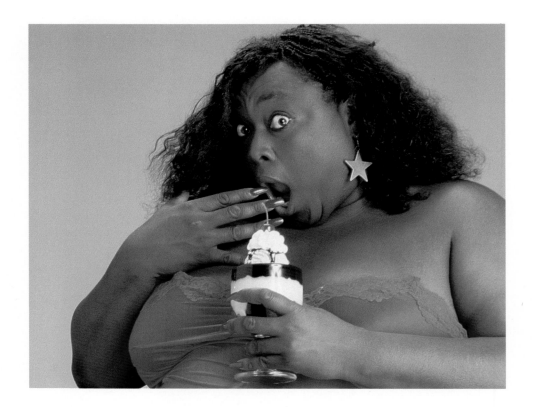

■ ICE CREAM

Ice cream is one of the first things some people give up on a diet. Honey, before I'd give up ice cream I'd give up breeding. And you know a womanthang like myself ain't about to give up breeding.

First of all, ice cream is made up of very healthy things—milk, eggs, and a little sugar ain't never hurt nobody either. Ice cream is high in calories and not something to be munched on like celery, but it won't get stuck between your teeth either, or make your tongue green.

It's just like with all the other goodies, if you deprive yourself of ice cream you'll end up feeling deprived and you won't be able to stay on your diet. So go ahead, honey, wrap those big lips around an Eskimo Pie and do it in the name of love.

■ CRACKERS & THANGS

Honey, believe me, you do not want me to start talking about "crackers and thangs." So let's just pass right by this obvious one and get right on to the calories in your favorite snack. Well, okay, your second favorite snack.

■ CHEESE

Now some of your more bionic diet experts will say that eating cheese is like thanking God for stretch pants. But I say that to deprive yourself of anything on a diet and expect it to be successful ultimately, is like waiting on Webster's Dictionary to be made into a movie. Self-destructive things, like overeating are based in denial and deprivation already, which is a whole other psychology essay that I don't have the time or the credentials to go into properly. But let's just say this. The "t" in dieting successfully is learning how to eat anything and everything you want and maintaining your desired weight. True, cheese is high in calories, but everything in life that's good is illegal, immoral, fattening or taxable, so what's a girl to do but throw her head back, act real white and strut right through it. So here's to brie on your breath, honey.

■ SOUPS

Soups are like love affairs, there ain't no tellin' what's in them. Not to mention everybody has their opinion of what makes a good one and what makes a bad one. And like the old saying goes, "too many cooks will spoil one in a hot minute." So how then can I propose to tell you how many calories are in a soup, or how many are in any given soup without having made it made it myself. So what I did was to decide how many calories would be in a basic type of typical soup. The only real way that you can tell how many calories are in a soup is if you count the calories of the components yourself. If you're seriously trying to lose weight I wouldn't advise eating a lot of soups because it is hard to count the calories unless, of course, you're toothless, in which case you must do what a girl has to do.

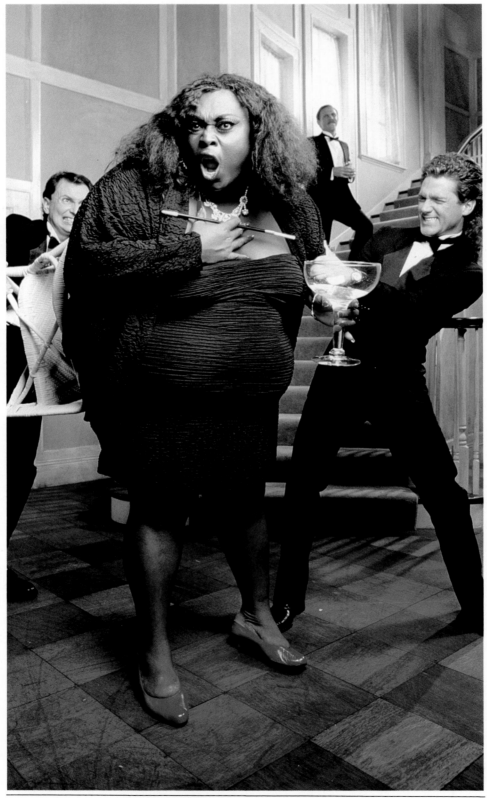

Sisters of Plenty Unite! Nuke Wicker!

□ WEIGHTS & MEASURES

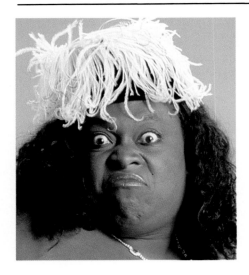

Honey, when it comes to talking about weight, the first thing that pops into my mind is that weight broke the bridge down and that's the whole issue here, i.e. the issue of the certain uncomfortabilities of being a Sister of Plenty.

For example there was the time that I was out to lunch in Hollywood with my acting class from Paramount. We had ordered our lunch and the drinks had arrived. I was a bit hung over, because I had gotten a tad embibed the night before. So I was drinking tomato juice, the only true hangover cure. Well just as I put the glass up to my mouth, the chair underneath me crumbled and I went sprawling all over the floor much to the shock and chagrin of this all too trendy Hollywood brunch crowd. The restaurant was totally silent. Then this little old Jewish lady of about 75 years or so, came running up to me with the largest, guadiest handbag in Hollywood, and said, "Sue, honey, sue! You're not that big, that chair should've held you. You're big, but you're not that big. You got a good law suit here." Then she started rambling through her bag and pulled out a beat up business card and said, "Here's my son's card. He's a lawyer and he'll be able to help you."

A week later, I was at this very well bred New York actress' garden Easter party in West Hollywood. They had little tiny white folding chairs, which I just knew would break. So I made a point of getting myself a special chair from Pamela's trendy apartment. It was a sturdy looking bamboo, cane and wicker number. Half way through the party the chair disintegrated underneath me and I fell into my date's potato salad, and turned over the table.

I went fleeing from the garden. Again, not a sound from the horrified, well bred crowd. Well, almost not a sound. A tacky little Ohio hussy, Josephine DeFrancis, who was conceived and born in the back seat of a pizza delivery truck, picked up a piece of the chair and came running behind me yelling, "Bev, Bev, you forgot your chair!" You see, she was after the man I was dating and thought this was the perfect time to humble me.

I went for a walk, that night after the party . . . me, a bottle of bourbon, and my fur. I hurt all over. I had been humiliated in front of my friends and the man I loved. As the bourbon went down, my anger rose, and it was not

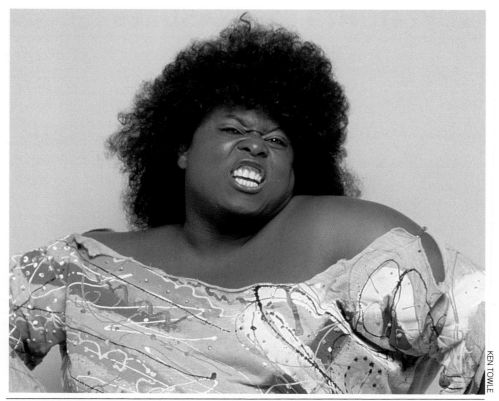

KEN TOWLE

Weight is like a man. Sometimes what seems like a little is a lot, and other times what seems like a lot ain't but a little.

long before I decided that Josephine De Francis had to be dealt with and in a cold blooded Detroit fashion.

To make a long story short, in a matter of two months, Josephine called me up on the phone and said, "You can have this man! You can have this town! I'm going back to New York City, I've had enough!" I said, "Bon voyage dahling and give my love to Bellevue." It's not important what I did, let's just say, I sank my fingernails into her crusty hope chest, and raked her up and down Hollywood Boulevard a couple of times . . . figuratively speaking, of course.

Now the point of all this is, that I have gained at least a hundred pounds since then and have not broken a single chair since. Now what does that tell you? It tells you that weight is a funny thang, so you have to be careful with it. Sometimes, what seems like a little is a lot, and other times what seems like a lot ain't but a little . . . as is the case with men.

So I have written this weights and measures chart for you, so you will have something to guide your food plan by. ■

WEIGHTS & MEASURES

UNIT	EQUIVALENT	METRIC EQUIVALENT
Ton	2000 pounds	.907 metric tons
hundredweight	100 pounds	45.359 kilograms
pound	16 ounces	.453 kilograms
ounce	16 drams	28.349 grams
dram	27.343 grains	1.771 grams
grain	.036 drams	.0648 grams
gallon	4 quarts	3.785 liters
quart	2 pints	.946 liters
pint	4 gills	.473 liters
gill	4 fluidounces	118.291 milliliters
fluidounce	8 fluidrams	25.573 milliliters
fluidram	60 minims	3.696 milliliters
minim	1/60 fluidram	.0061610 milliliters
bushel	4 pecks	35.238 liters
peck	8 quarts	8.809 liters
mile	5,280 feet	1,609 kilometers
rod	5.50 yards	5,029 meters
yard	3 feet	.9144 meters
foot	12 inches	30.480 centimeters
inch	.093 feet	2.540 centimeters
square mile	640 acres	2.590 sq. kilometers
acre	4840 square	.405 hectares
square rod	30.25 square yards	25.293 square meters
square yard	1296 square inches	.836 square meters
square foot	144 square inches	.093 square meters
square inch	.007 square feet	6.45 square cm
cubic yard	27 cubic feet	.765 cubic meters
cubic foot	1728 cubic inches	.028 cubic meters
cubic inch	.00058 cubic feet	16.387 cubic cm
1 bolopa	2 thangs	none
1 thang	2 thingies	none
1 thingy	2 thingomajiggies	none
1 thingomajiggy	2 doohickies	none
1 doohicky	2 doodads	Ricardo Montebaln
1 doodad	2 dribblins	none
1 dribblin	2 duncanettes	none
1 duncanette	2 suckas	none
1 sucka	2 smackins	none
1 smackin	2 crustettes	none
1 crustette	3 scrunchettes	none
1 scrunchette	2 tads	none
1 tad	4 tadlettes	none
1 tadlette	2 smidgens	none
1 smidgen	1/2 of a tadlette	none

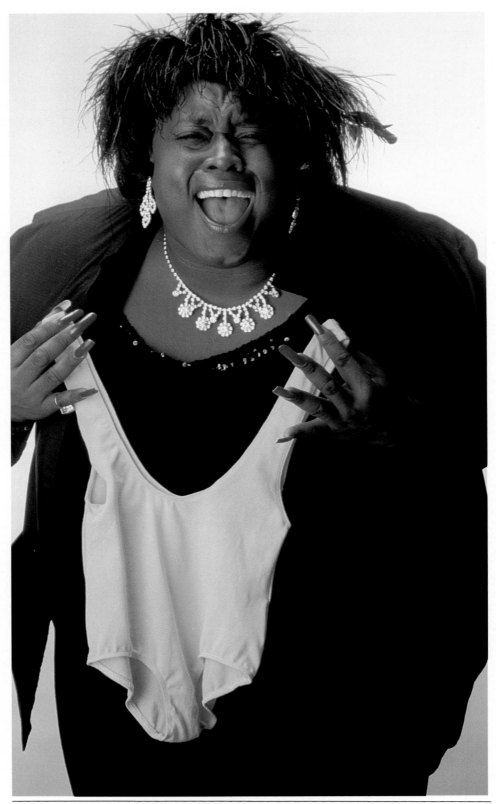

I've got will power. It's won't power that I'm low on.

□ **WILL POWER**

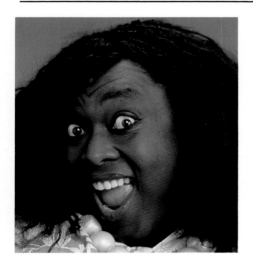

It's really not even the issue of will power that we need to discuss, because it's actually not will power that one needs when trying to lose weight. It's *won't* power.

"Won't power," as in "No, I won't go to the Donut Hole and have four dozen bear claws at 4:00 A.M." Won't power, as in "No, I won't order three large combination pizzas and a bucket of chicken."

I used to think that if will power were tits I'd be a Chinese girl. Then I realized that I actually have a lot of will power. Let me decide that I want to have something to munch on at any hour of the night in any town, in any foodless home, during any monsoon, twister or blizzard, and you'll see exactly how much will power I have. Most Sisters of Plenty are the same. Most uf us have *plenty* of will power.

So again, the question is, as I stated at the beginning of this book: Do you really *want* to lose weight?

Now you might sincerely say yes, and believe that you do, and still know that the minute you put this book down you are going to go clean out your refrigerator, vacuum your cupboards, and then call Chicken Delight for a delivery.

So what do you do? Any diet book can give you a food plan that will work, but how many of them can help you stick to your plan? Where are they at 3:00 A.M. when you're eating English muffins like they're M&Ms? Know what I mean?

Now, I don't profess to be a psychologist or an expert, and technically I don't hold any of the degrees the government might require to be considered an authority on this subject.

However, I have been trying to lose weight ever since I was eight years old, and now I'm somewhere between Brooke Shields and death. I have tried all of the powders, all of the plans, all of the scams, hypnosis, acupuncture, injections, balloons, surgeries, all of them, and none of them have worked. And for one simple reason: I could not control my eating.

Now, this is what I have learned in my experience. Most people I have encountered who are overeaters like myself are individuals who have been kicked around in life, and usually in their early years. At some point they learned that when it hurts, the act of eating makes it feel better. Some of us are very angry, but anger is just the lid on sorrow, and the bottom line is that most of us are crying inside and trying to wipe those tears away with food.

So what you really have to do, and it's so scary, is sit down and find out what it is that is making you cry. Then you have to decide if that thing is so terrible that it's worth being fat over. If it is, then carry on. If it isn't, you have to come to terms with those feelings. Then you are ready.

You know, Mamma used to say, "A habit is a cable and each day it weaves a thread, until at last it is so strong you can't break it." That's so true with the habit of eating because of emotional feelings. What you have to do is unwind the cable, thread by thread, until it's weak enough for you to break it.

The way you unwind it is simple. Compulsive overeating is a learned behavior. And like any learned behavior it can be unlearned, or replaced by a different learned behavior. The emotional dysfunction in compulsive overeating is a lack of discipline. So in order to deal with the surface of the problem—the excess weight itself—the immediate issue is teaching yourself discipline.

While teaching yourself discipline will help you with the immediate problem of the weight, it is not the immediate problem that is the real problem, and that is what must be dealt with. Your task is to find another way in which to deal with the feelings. Some other ways are getting involved in a support group, individual or group therapy, or any number of other behavior modification programs. Such behavior modification programs might be something as simple as knitting when you're bored, as opposed to eating linguini like it's going out of style. Jogging to release frustration is another way, but you already know how I feel about *that* activity. The key to the whole program is fearless honesty. And the lock that must be opened is how you really *feel*. Only you know what is the most appropriate behavior modification system for yourself. So listen to the ultimate authority: yourself, and God, but not necessarily in that order.

Make it easy for yourself. Start by creating a simple system. Whatever is the easiest for you to adhere to at the time. When I started doing this, my regimen became anything I wanted as long as I didn't eat so much it made me throw up. I've progressed from there to three meals a day with nothing in between, and soon I will turn those three meals into three very light and healthy meals. But the bottom line is that I eat anything I want, and for the first time in my life I'm enjoying my food and losing weight, and not feeling the least bit deprived.

When you break your abstinence—and you will, because life is that way—it's just like when you get a new set of crystal glasses. They're wonderful and you're real careful with them, and you swear you'll never break one, and you look at them six months down the line and there's only three left. The same is true of sane eating, it's like any other diet. We start out like gangbusters, but end up signing off like "we the people." But this is not like any other diet in the respect that it's not a *diet*, it's a new way of *living*. It's just a change, like a change in your hair color or style of dress. And because this is not a diet, it's a change, when you break your abstinence it's no big deal. Just smooth your petticoats, blame it on the wind, and get back to your regimen. Don't feel guilty, don't blame yourself, just do as grandma used to do when the biscuits didn't turn out quite right. Throw your head back and say, "It be this a way sometimes," then get on to the gravy and peas. We are human beings, we are not perfect, and sometimes we're gonna make mistakes and do things we wish we hadn't. When you do slip, however, examine the circumstances closely and make sure you understand why. Understanding yourself and your surroundings is the key to your success.

Also, you must rebuild years of eroded self-esteem. That, too, is a simple process. Just start thinking about what things would make you feel better about yourself. Start being good to yourself in this way, just with little things, and easy things for you to do. The key here is "slow and steady, nice and easy." That'll win the race.

I know you want it yesterday. I do too. We all do. I'm still big enough to sell shade at parades but I'm on the happy road to losing weight, and I just walk that road one step at a time. If it were an instant thing, Kodak would've packaged it and it would be on the shelf next to the rest of the "miracle cures," and you wouldn't be reading this book and I wouldn't have written it. Remember that when the road looks long.

I don't mean to turn a humor book into something serious, heavy and spiritual, but laughter is the flip side of sorrow, and the fact is, obesity is a deadly disease and that's not a laughing matter. So every now and again even I, jester extraordinaire, must trudge the serious vein.

If you take only one thought from this book, please take this one: Listen closely to your laughter and your tears, for they are minstrels that come from your soul, and your soul is a gypsy dancing to the mandolin of your experience. To turn a deaf ear is to deny life itself. If you understand that, someday you'll understand why this is ... the *last* diet book. ∎

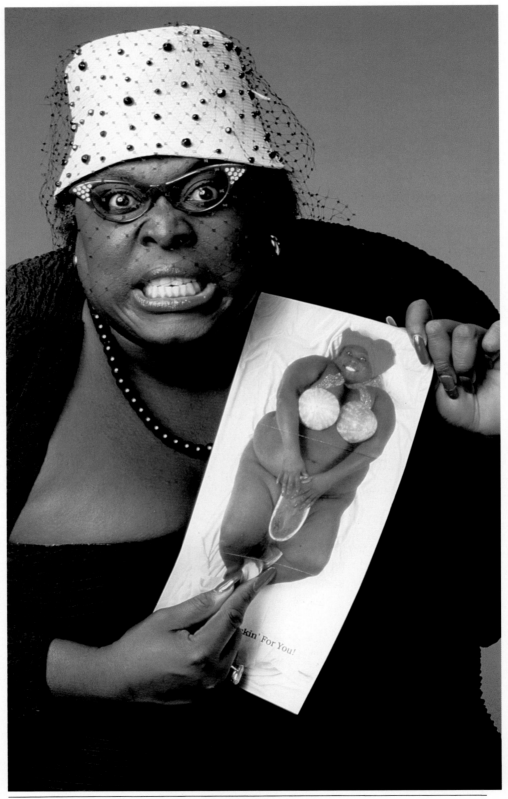

We are not amused.

☐ GLOSSARY

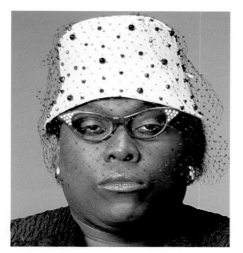

I know it seems strange that one would include a glossary with a diet book. Trust me, stranger things are being done, and probably right in your building or for sure on your block.

I have included a glossary, because a Sister of Plenty is a very unique and special blossom in the garden of life and thus requires special and unique terms. Terms that relate to the specific, unique nature of her encounters.

The other reason I have included a glossary is that I just don't have the time to deal with the phone calls from you sheltered heifers across the country calling me up, giving me the flux in the middle of the day, trying to find out what I'm talking about because I'm speaking in the tongue of the 80's.

I'm dead serious, honey, I have got sales to attend. This is rummage sale season, and I've got better things to do. That's right, you heard me correctly. Child, Sister Fung Pung, of the "Sisters of Sappho in Sumo Wrestling" is having her annual used Kimono sale, and I could use some new kimonos. And God knows that's a sale that you're gonna have to get to early, nothing is more dangerous than a bevy of heavies trying to fight their way to a bargain. The body heat alone is enough to ruin a girl's perm. Not to mention once those girls get to steppin' and fetchin' and carryin' on it gets down right criminally dangerous.

Besides the economic and health aspects of this rummage sale, there is also the social aspect. That's right, not only does Sister Pung have a kimono sale but she also has a jacuzzi and pool party. Well, this year it's gonna be just a pool party because the jacuzzi was destroyed last year, accidently.

You see the jacuzzi was about 8 feet off of the ground in a redwood deck. Well, on the side of the hot tub itself, it said maximum capacity 12 persons. Honey, 8 of the Sisters of Plenty got up into that tub and she broke off at the fixtures and went crashing to the ground. Well, natually when that happened, there was no more temperature control on the water, so the scalding hot water was tearing those Sisters of Plenty's behinds up. It was not pretty. No, let me rephrase that. It was ugly. We're talking shake and bake. The worse thing about it was that the Sisters of Plenty weren't strong enough to pull themselves up and out of the hole. Finally, they had to call the fire department. Well, these little skinny firemen couldn't pull these big womanthangs out either. So they had to chop a hole in the side of the deck and let the good times roll, so to speak.

Now do you see what I mean? Cause honey, I was in that jacuzzi. What if you had been calling me up at that time to find out the meaning of a word? When I did get to the phone, I would not have been in the mood. So, that my dear, is why there is a glossary.

Bolopa	1. A unit of measure used in dieting by the trendy. 2. A Polish Mistress.
Thang	1. A unit of measure; two thingies. 2. A one-eyed, purpled-veined, moisture-seeking wand of destruction.
Thingy	1. A one-eyed, purple-veined, moisture-seeking, wand of no consequence. 2. A small unit of measure.
Doohicky	1. Love mark left by Loretta Lynn's husband. 2. Two doodads.
Dribblin	1. A trait negro children are born with in their hands. 2. A unit of measure usually used in determining a quantity of cornbread.
Duncanette	1. Child of Sandy Duncan. 2. Anybody who eats more than one Wheat Thin. 3. A unit of measure.
Coos Coos	1. Arabic dish. 2. A Creole hooker. 3. Female Platypus gentalia
Sucka	1. Male population of Detroit. 2. A unit of measure: 2 smackins
Smackin	1. Minority child development technique 2. 2 crustettes.
Tad	1. 4 tadlettes. 2. A cute boy on *All My Children* who has married Hilary, and is now working at the bank and trying to be good, after sleeping with every woman in Pine Valley except Mrs. Guerney and Myra Sloan.
Sailor	1. Something God invented to deal with the rent.
Doodad	1. Elderly straight male hairdresser. 2. Unit of measure; 2 dribblins.
Thingomajiggy	1. Small unit of measure: 1/2 of a thingy. 2. Oriental reproductive organ.
Tadlette	1. A black girl from Gary, Indiana that used to beat Michael Jackson up. 2. Two smidgens.

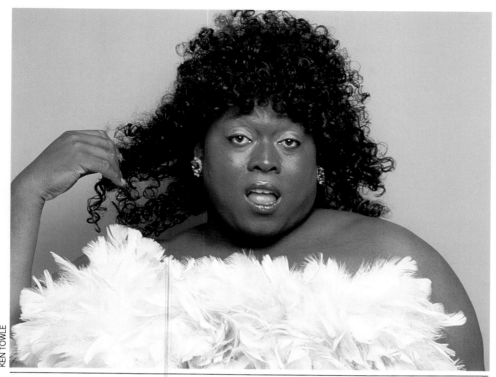

KEN TOWLE

The answer is yes. Now, what's the question?

Scrunchette
1. Tadlette's big sister.
2. Things they remove from white women during corrective surgery.
3. A unit of measure: 2 tads.

Piggly Wiggly
1. A chain of southern grocery stores.
2. A Sister of Plenty doing the shimmy.
3. A small cute pig who saved an Irish family from ruin.

Hogly Wogly
1. Piggly Wiggly's mammy.

Democrat
1. People who believe in withdrawal as a viable means of birth control.

Republican
1. Someone whose God is profit and fuel for living is greed.
2. Someone who had the American Dream come true.

Smidgen
1. A Latvian midget who manages prostitutes.
2. With the exception of Dolly Parton, any white woman's tit.

Ricardo Montebalm
1. The reason silent film Divas go on living.
2. A reason to look "marvelous".

Gourds
1. Things white women with coffee colored spots on their hands put in the center of their tables at Thanksgiving.
2. Things Mexican housekeepers dust.

Creekin'
1. A term negroes use.

GAP
1. Gay American Princess.
2. Someone who could suck a cantelope through the eye of a sewing needle.
3. Citizen of West Hollywood.

West Hollywood
1. Swish Alps.
2. City whose major crime is breaking, entering and redecorating.

Blow Dryer
1. Official bird of West Hollywood.
2. Official animal of West Hollywood.
3. Official flower of West Hollywood.

Macon
1. City in Georgia.
2. Cured meat from a Wart Hog that is usually served at breakfast in tribal communities.

Detail Nazi
1. Someone who would wipe the water spots off the Golden Gate Bridge before photographing it.
2. Randal "Wait, there's a piece of lint in her hair" West.

Austin
1. City where men are men, and women are grateful.

San Francisco
1. A city where men are men and women are out of luck.

Los Angeles
1. City where men are men and women are too.

East Los Angeles
1. The capital of Mexico.
2. The reason Chevrolets are still on the market.

Exercise
1. Vigorous use of the body to try and stay in shape.
2. Any physical action more difficult than breathing.

Calorie
1. The amount of heat required at the pressure of one atmosphere to raise the temperature of one gram of water, one degree Celsius.
2. The ruin of many a good girl.

Diet
1. A food plan.
2. A small "Di".

Starch
1. The main ingredient in the upper lip of a WASP.
2. High carbohydrate substance that is avoided on diets a great deal.

Protein
1. A substance made by the synthesis of amino acids.
2. A black girl in Niles, Michigan.

Carbohydrates
1. Neutral compounds of carbons, hydrogens and oxygens.
2. A process of freeze-drying carburetors to smuggle them across the Mexican border.

Fat
1. Animal tissue filled with greasy or oily matter.
2. Something God made to prevent people from wearing their lips and gums out prematurely.

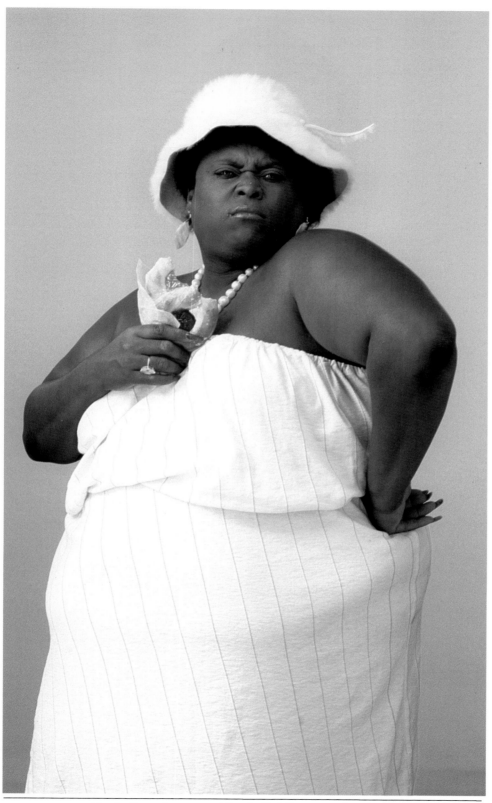

Yeah, there's a word for it. But they won't print it.

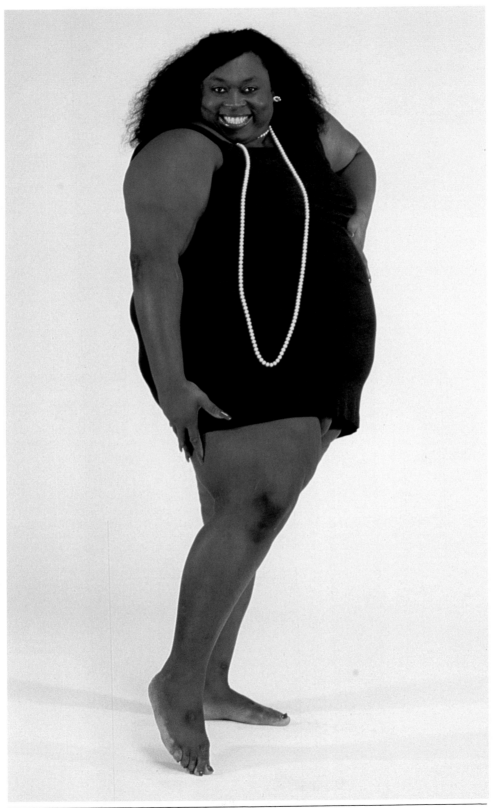

Same old body. Same old dress. But a new attitude.

MEAT

	Amt*	Cal		Amt*	Cal
BEEF	1		Beef (jellied)	1**	45
Brisket	1	63	Gourmet Loaf	1	35
Chuck	1	93	Ham Roll	1**	43
Filet Mignon	1	63	Honey Loaf	1**	40
Flank	1	56	Iowa Brand	1**	45
Foreshank	1	78	Liver Cheese	1**	113
Ground (lean)	1	62	Liver Loaf	1**	40
Hamburger	1	81	Luxury Loaf	1**	39
Heal of Round	1	74	Macaroni & Cheese Loaf	1**	70
Hindshank	1	102	New England Sausage	1**	35
Neck	1	83	Old Fashioned Loaf	1**	70
Plate	1	135	Olive Loaf	1**	80
Rib Roast	1	125	Peppered Loaf	1**	40
Round	1	74	Pickle Loaf	1**	80
Rump	1	98	Pickle & Pimento Loaf	1**	65
Steak, Club	1	129	Spiced Loaf	1**	75
Steak, Porterhouse	1	132	Salami	1**	128
Steak, Ribeye	1	125	LAMB		
Steak, Sirloin, double-bone	1	116	Chop, loin	1	100
Steak, sirloin, hipbone	1	138	Chop, rib	1	115
Steak, sirloin, wedge & round bone	1	110	Leg	1	79
Steak, T-Bone	1	134	Shoulder	1	96
PORK			Lamb's Quarter	1	9
Boston butt	1	100	VARMITS		
Chop	1	83	Rabbit	1	61
Ham	1	75	Raccoon	1	63
Loin	1	103	Opossum	1	62
Picnic	1	106	Squirrel	1	60
Spare Ribs	1	125	Muskrat	1	43
VEAL			OBSCURE PARTS		
Chuck	1	67	Liver, Beef	1	65
Flank	1	115	Liver, Calf	1	74
Foreshank	1	61	Liver, Hog	1	68
Loin	1	66	Liver, Lamb	1	39
Plate	1	86	Lung, Beef	1	27
Rib	1	45	Lung, Calf	1	30
Round & Rump	1	76	Lung, Lamb	1	29
Steak, Cutlet	1	61	Pancreas, Beef	1	40
LUNCHEON MEATS			Pancreas, Calf	1	46
Bologna	1**	98	Sweetbread, Hog	1	69
Banquet Loaf	1**	50	Stomach, Pork (Hog Mawl)	1	43
Barbecue Loaf	1**	43	Chitterlings (Chit'lins)	1	64

*OUNCE   **SLICE

RED MEAT THANGS

	Amt*	Cal		Amt*	Cal
Bacon	1**	43	Pastrami	1	47
Canadian Bacon	1	61	Potted Meat	1	50
Corned Beef	1	106	Pigs Feet	1	25
Beef Jerky	1	85	Pepperoni	1	140
Corned Beef Spread	1	70	Prosciutto	1	90
Braunschweiger	1	80	Salt Pork (Fat Back)	1	222
Roast Beef Spread	1	62	Spam	1	85
Mincemeat	1	100	Sausage, Brown 'n Serve	1	120
Tongue, Beef	1	69	Sausage, Patty	1	150
Tongue, Calf	1	45	Sausage, Polish	1	95
Tongue, Hog	1	72	Sausage, Kolbase	1	107
Tongue, Lamb	1	72	Sausage, Kolbasa	1	94
Tongue, Sheep	1	92	Sausage, Beef	1	112
Sizzlelean	1	50	Sausage, Smokey Link	1 Lnk	70
Head Cheese	1	76	Sausage, Rolled	1	80
Hotdogs	1	140	Sausage, Smoked	1	95

*OUNCE   **SLICE

BREAD

	Amt	Cal		Amt	Cal
Apple Cinnamon	1	70	Multi-Grain	1	35
Boston Brown	1	101	Oat	1	110
Corn & Molasses	1	75	Oatmeal	1	70
Cracked Wheat	1	75	Onion (party size)	1	15
Crispbread, Mora	1	333	Orange & Raisin	1	70
Crispbread, Rye	1	37	Protein	1	45
Crispbread, Sesame	1	50	Pumpernickel	1	85
Date Nut Roll	1	80	Raisin	1	80
Date Walnut	1	75	Rye	1	80
Flatbread, Bran	1	19	Salt Rising	1	67
Flatbread, Thin	1	12	Z-Grain	1	72
French	1	80	Sourdough	1	70
Hillbilly	1	72	Sprouted Wheat	1	65
Hollywood	1	72	Vienna	1	75
Honey Bran	1	95	Cracked Wheat	1	105
Honey Wheat Berry	1	90	White	1	65
Italian	1	70	Buttermilk White	1	75
Low Sodium	1	71	Whole Wheat	1	60

FAST FOOD

	Amt	Cal		Amt	Cal
Arby's Bacon Cheddar Dix	1	560	Double Beef Whopper	1	740
Arby's Beef & Cheddar	1	450	Double Beef Whooper w/cheese	1	950
Arby's French Dip	1	386	McDonald's Big Mac	1	563
Arby's Ham & Cheese	1	380	White Castle Hamburger	1	160
Arby's Regular R.B.	1	350			

VEGETABLES, LEGUMES & THANGS

	Amt	Cal		Amt	Cal
Barley	1	99	Bibb Lettuce	1	3
Black Beans	1	103	Boston Lettuce	1	3
Garbanzo Beans	1	105	Grand Rapids Lettuce	1	3
Artichoke	1	12	Great Lakes Lettuce	1	4
Asparagus	1	4	New York Lettuce	1	4
Avocado	1	47	Romaine Lettuce	1	3
Green Beans	1	7	Salad Bowl Lettuce	1	3
Kidney Beans	1	97	Simpson Lettuce	1	3
Lima Beans	1	97	White Paris Lettuce	1	4
Mung Beans	1	96	Mushroom	1	9
Pinto Beans	1	99	Chinese Mushroom	1	80
Bean Sprouts	1	13	Mustard Greens	1	7
Wax Beans	1	7	New Zealand Spinach	1	4
Beets	1	12	Okra	1	10
Broccoli	1	7	Olive	1	96
Bulgar	1	100	Onion	1	10
Cabbage	1	7	Parsley	1	13
Carrots	1	12	Parsnip	1	19
Cauliflower	1	8	Green Peas	1	20
Celery	1	5	Black-eyed Peas	1	35
Chard	1	7	June Peas	1	35
Chick Peas	1	105	Pea Pods	1	12
Collard Greens	1	9	Green Pepper	1	8
Corn	1	24	Potato	1	23
Cucumber	1	4	Rhubarb	1	23
French Fries	1	100	Brown Rice	1	30
Dandelion Greens	1	9	White Rice	1	31
Egg Plant	1	5	Rutabaga	1	13
Endive	1	6	Sauerkraut	1	5
Escarole	1	6	Agar Seaweed	1	90
Farina	1	96	Lavar Seaweed	1	70
Jerusalem Artichoke	1	19	Soybeans	1	36
Kale	1	11	Spinach	1	7
Leeks	1	15	Summer Squash	1	4
Lentils	1	97	Acorn Squash	1	19
			Sweet Potato	1	40
			Tomato	1	7
			Turnips	1	9
			Turnip Greens	1	7
			Wax Gourds		

Thanksgiving Centerpieces;
don't even think about putting
them in your mouth.

YOGURT

	Amt	Cal		Amt	Cal
Plain	8 oz	160	Date Walnut Raisin	8 oz	260
Apple	8 oz	260	Fruit Crunch	8 oz	210
Banana	8 oz	260	Granola Strawberry	8 oz	240
Banana-Strawberry	8 oz	235	Guava	8 oz	240
Blueberry	8 oz	260	Hawaiian Salad	8 oz	210
Boysenberry	8 oz	260	Honey Vanilla	8 oz	220
Cherry	8 oz	260	Lemon	8 oz	200
Cherry-Vanilla	8 oz	250	Orange	8 oz	210
Coffee	8 oz	200	Peach	8 oz	260

FRUIT

	Amt	Cal
Apple	1 med	60
Apricot	1	14
Banana	1	17
Balsampear	1	5
Blackberry	1	16
Blueberry	1	16
Boysenberry	1	16
Cantelope	1	8
Casaba Melon	1	8
Sweet Cherries	1	71
Sour Cherries	1	60
Coconut	1	98
Cranberry	1	13
Currant	1	15
Date	1	77
Elderberry	1	20
Fig	1	26
Fruit Cocktail	1	17
Grape	1	12
Grapefruit	1/2 med	50
Guava	1	18
Honeydew	1	9
Jackfruit	1	26
Jujube	1	30
Kumquat	1	18
Lemon	1	8
Lime	1	8
Mango	1	13
Nectarine	1	10
Orange	1	11
Passion Fruit	1	13
Peach	1	9
Pear	1	7
Persimmon	1	36
Pineapple	1	15
Plum	1	34
Pomegranate	1	17
Prickly Pear	1	12
Prune	1	60
Pumpkin	1	157
Raisin	1	90
Raspberry	1	20
Strawberry	1	10
Tangelo	1	26
Tangerine	1	10
Watermelon	1	4

POULTRY

	Amt	Cal
Arby's Chicken Sandwich	1	584
Chicken	1	39
Chicken Pie	1	520
Potted Chicken	1	70
Dairy Queen Chicken Sandwich	1	670
Domestic Duck	1	47
Wild Duck	1	39
Egg White	1 lg	17
Egg Yolk	1 lg	59
Goose	1	86
Goose Gizzard	1	38
Goose Liver	1	47
Mc Donald's Chicken McNuggets	6 pcs	314
SAUCES:		
Barbecue	1	60
Honey	1	50
Honey Mustard	1	63
Sweet & Sour	1	64
Guinea Hen	1	44
Ponderosa Chicken Strips	1 ordr	282
Pheasant	1	46
Quail	1	49
Squab	1	42
Turkey, Dark Meat	1	36
Turkey, Light Meat	1	33
Turkey Franks	1	95
Turkey Salami	1 sli	50
Turkey Bologna	1 sli	60
Turkey Ham	1 sli	45
Turkey Pie	1	526
Turkey Gizzards	1 thingy	56
Potted Turkey	1	70

Turkey Liver
Turkey's don't have livers.
(Think about it. Have you ever met a turkey that wasn't a drunk?)

FISH

	Amt	Cal
Abalone	1	38
Albacore	1	50
Anchovy	1	40
Black Sea Bass	1	22
Large Fresh Water Bass	1	25
Bluefish	1	32
Bonito	1	48
Buffalo Fish	1	31
Butterfish (Northern)	1	48
Butterfish (Gulf)	1	27
Carp	1	31
Catfish	1	29
Caviar	1 tbs	42
Clams	1	23
Mrs. Paul's Fried Clams	1	92
Clam Juice	1	30
Cod	1	22
Crab	1	26
Mrs. Paul's Fried Crab	6 oz	340
Croaker	1	27
Raw Eel	1	94
Smoked Eel	1	67
Flounder	1	23
Gefilte Fish	1	15
Grouper	1	25
Haddock	1	23
Halibut	1	21
Smoked Halibut	1	64
Jack Mackerel	1	41
Kingfish	1	30
Lake Herring	1	26
Lake Trout	1	24
Lingcod	1	22
Mullet	1	28
Muskellunge	1	34
Mussels	1	22

	Amt*	Cal
Octopus	1	21
Oyster	1	54
Pike	1	25
Red Snapper	1	21
Roe	1	58
Sablefish	1	53
Salmon:		
Atlantic	1	61
Chinook	1	63
Pink	1	31
Sockeye	1	46
Smoked	1	50
Sardines in Oil	3¾	330
Sardines in Mustard	3¾	230
Sardines in Tomato	3¾	230
Scallops	1	32
Sea Bass	1	23
Shad	1	48
Shrimp	1	26
Smelt	1	27
Snail (Escargot)	1	25
Sole	1	22
Spanish Mackerel	1	25
Squid	1	23
Sturgeon	1	26
Smoked Sturgeon	1	42
Sucker	1	31
Swordfish	1	33
Tautug	1	25
Tuna (Raw)	1	41
Tuna in Oil	1	106
Tuna in Water	1	52
Turbot	1	41
Turtle (Green Sea)	1	25
Turtle (Snapping)	1	42
Whitefish	1	44

FISH THANGS

	Amt	Cal
McDonald's Filet-o-Fish	1**	432
White Castle Fishwich	1**	192
Mrs. Paul's Fish Sticks	1	58

*Ounces

**Sandwich

SOUPS

	Amt*	Cal		Amt*	Cal
Cream of Shrimp	8	160	Cream of Onion	8	160
Chunky Sirloin Burger	8	165	Oyster Stew	8	140
Chunky Steak & Potato	8	123	Green Pea	8	150
Tomato	8	90	Chunky Split Pea & Ham	8	167
Tomato Bisque	8	120	Split Pea, Ham		
Garden Tomato	8	80	& Bacon	8	170
Old Fashioned			Pepper Pot	8	90
Tomato & Rice	8	110	Cream of Potato	8	130
Turkey Noodle	8	60	Scotch Broth	8	80
Turkey Vegetable	8	70	Cream of Asparagus	8	90
Chunky Vegetable	8	112	Chunky Ham & Bean	8	214
Chunky Old Fashioned	8	120	Black Bean	8	110
Beef Vegetable	8	70	Chunky Beef	8	123
Old Fashioned Vegetable	8	60	Chunky Beef		
Vegetarian Vegetable	8	70	With Noodles	8	217
Vichyssoise	8	85	Broth (Plain)	8	16
Won Ton	8	40	Broth & Barley	8	60
Chicken Noodle O's	8	70	Broth & Noodles	8	60
Chicken & Rice	8	60	Consomme	8	25
Chicken & Stars	8	50	Mushroom Broth	8	70
Chicken Vegetable	8	70	Noodle Broth	8	70
Chunky Chili Beef	8	217	Teriyaki Broth	8	70
Chunky Manhattan			Cream of Celery	8	100
Clam Chowder	8	116	Cheddar Cheese	8	130
Manhattan Clam Chowder	8	70	Chunky Chicken	8	125
New England			Old Fashioned Chicken		
Clam Chowder	8	150	and Rice (Chunky)	8	120
Gazpacho	8	50	Chunky Chicken Vegetable	8	160
Minestrone	8	80	Chicken & Alphabet	8	80
Cream of Mushroom	8	100	Chicken Broth (Plain)	8	35
Golden Mushroom	8	80	Chicken Broth & Rice	8	50
Mushroom Barley	8	80	Chicken Broth & Vegetable	8	25
Curly Noodle & Chicken	8	70	Cream of Chicken	8	110
Curly Noodle &			Chicken & Dumplings	8	90
Ground Beef	8	90	Chicken Gumbo	8	60
Onion	8	70	Creamy Chicken Mushroom	8	110
			Chicken Noodle	8	70

ICE CREAM

	Amt*	Cal		Amt*	Cal
Butter Pecan	1	32	Rocky Road	1	88
Black Cherry	1	38	Tin Roof	1	65
Chocolate	1	66	Blue Moon	1	45
Chocolate Chip	1	38	Neopolitan	1	47
Eskimo Pie	1 bar	180	Double Fudge Nut	1	85
Fudge Royal	1	30	Jamocha Almond Fudge	1	77
Peach	1	32	Cappucino	1	55
Pralines-N-Cream	1	44	Danish Nut Roll	1	45
Strawberry	1	56	Chocolate Chip Mint	1	58
Toffee Fudge Swirl	1	45	Ice Cream Cone	1	20
Vanilla	1	32			
Blueberry Cheesecake	1	55			

CHEESE

	Amt*	Cal		Amt*	Cal
American	1	105	Limburger	1	93
Blue Cheese	1	104	Longhorn	1	106
Bonbino Natural	1	100	Meunster	1	104
Brick	1	105	Monterey Jack	1	100
Brie*	1	80	Mozzarella	1	90
Camembert	1	85	Nibblin Curds	1	113
Colby	1	110	Parmesan Grated	1	50
Cottage Cheese	1	65	Parmesan Whole	1	110
Cream Cheese	1	106	French Pot Cheese	1	30
Edam	1	100	Provalone	1	100
Farmers	1	86	Ricotta	1	40
Feta	1	76	Romano	1	110
Gjetost Norwegian	1	118	Roquefort	1	104
Gouda	1	100	Samsoe Danish	1	100
Gruyere	1	100	Scamorze	1	79
Havarti	1	90	Stirred Curd	1	110
Hoop Natural	1	21	String Cheese	1	90
Jalapeno Pepper Cheese	1	112	Swiss Cheese	1	105
Jarlsberg Norwegian	1	100	Washed Curd	1	108
Kettle Moraine	1	100			

CHEESE THANGS

	Amt*	Cal
Snack Mate (Nabisco)	1	64
Velveeta	1	85
Cheese Whiz	1	78
Weight Watchers	1	50
Cheese Flavored Puffs	1	210

*Ounces

COOKIES

	Amt	Cal		Amt	Cal
Almond Windmill	1	47	Lemon Nut	1	57
Animal Cracker	1	11	Lido	1	95
Apple	1	50	Marshmallow Sandwich	1	30
Apple Crisp	1	50	Marshmallow Banana	1	127
Apple Spice	1	55	Milano	1	60
Apricot Raspberry	1	49	Milano Mint	1	76
Bordeaux	1	33	Molasses	1	60
Brown Edge Wafer	1	28	Molasses Crisp	1	33
Brownie	1	251	Nassau	1	85
Brussles	1	55	Nilla Wafer	1	19
Brussles Mint	1	67	Oreo	1	50
Butter	1	23	Oatmeal (plain)	1	47
Buttercup	1	25	Oatmeal Raisin	1	57
Butterscotch Chip	1	80	Orange Milano	1	76
Cappucino	1	53	Orleans	1	30
Capri	1	80	Orleans Sandwich	1	60
Caramel Peanut Log	1	120	Peanut Butter	1	47
Chessman	1	43	Pecan Sandies	1	86
Chocolate Fudge Strip	1	54	Pecan Icebox	1	48
Chocolate Pinwheel	1	140	Piccolo	1	22
Chocolate Snap	1	16	Raisin	1	107
Chocolate Chip	1	85	Raisin Fruit Biscuit	1	60
Chocolate Peanut Bar	1	95	Iced Raisin Bar	1	80
Cinnamon Sugar	1	53	Raisin Bran Cookie	1	53
Coconut Bar	1	43	Creme Sandwich	1	83
Coconut Macaroon	1	96	Shortbread	1	7
Coconut Chocolate Drop	1	87	Shortbread-Lorna Doone	1	40
Coconut Granola	1	57	Social Tea Biscuit	1	22
Coconut Creme Stick	1	39	Spiced Wafer	1	33
Date Nut Granola	1	53	Spiced Windmill	1	60
Date Pecan	1	53	St. Moritz	1	57
Fig Newton	1	60	Strawberry	1	50
Geneva	1	57	Sugar	1	50
Gingerman	1	33	Sugar Wafer	1	36
Gingersnap	1	32	Sunflower Raisin	1	53
Granola	1	120	Tahiti	1	85
Hazelnut	1	57	Waffle Creme	1	45
Ladyfinger	1	40	Zanzibar	1	40

CRACKERS & THANGS

	Amt	Cal
American Harvest	1 doohicky	16
Arrowroot Biscuit	1 doohicky	20
Bacon 'n Dip	1 doohicky	9
Bacon-flavored Thins	1 doohicky	11
Bacon Nips	Smidgen	147
Biscos	1 doohicky	19
Bran Wafer	1 tadlette	13
Bugles	Smidgen	150
Cheese Bops	1 tadlette	147
Cheetos	1 tad	160
Cornponettes	1 dribblin	160
Chicken In a Biskit	1 doohicky	11
Chippers	1 doohicky	15
Chipsters	1 doohicky	2
Club Cracker	1 doohicky	15
Fritos, Regular	1 dribblin	160
Fritos, Barbecue	1 dribblin	150
Flings	1 doohicky	10
Goldfish	1 doohicky	10
Graham Cracker	1 doohicky	30
Graham, Chocolate Covered	1 doohicky	65
Korkers	1 doohicky	8
Meal Mates	1 thingy	22
Onion	1 doohicky	15
Oyster	1 scrunchette	3
Pumpernickel Toast	1 doohicky	15
Ritz	1 doohicky	17
Rich & Crisp	1 doohicky	14
Roman Meal Wafer	1 doohicky	11
Royal Lunch	1 scrunchette	55
Rusk, Holland	1 thingy	40
Rye Krisp	1 doodad	30
Saltine	1 thingy	12
Sea Rounds	1 doodad	45
Sesame	1 thingy	12
Shindigs	1 bolopa	6
Snaks Ahoy	1 bolopa	9
Tortilla Chips	Honey, Please	
Townhouse Cracker	1 doodad	16
Triscuit	1 thingy	20
Twiddle Sticks	1 bolopa	53
Twigs	1 twig	14
Uneeda Biscuit	No you don't	
Vergetable Thin	1 vegee	12
Waldorf	1 crustette	12
Waverly Wafer	1 smidgen	18
Wheat Chips	1 bolopa	4
Wheat Thin	1 Duncanette	10

CANDY

	Amt	Cal		Amt	Cal
Almond, Chocolate Coated	1 oz	161	Lollipop	1 pop	100
Butterscotch	1 oz	115	Mallo Cup	1 doohicky	54
Candy Corn	1 oz	100	Milk Duds	1 oz	100
Caramel	1 oz	120	Milkyway	1 bar	267
Chocolate, Milk	1 oz	150	Mr. Goodbar	1 bar	54
Coconut Bon Bons	1 oz	125	Nestle's $100,000	1 bar	175
Fondant	1 oz	100	Orange Slices	1 sli	30
Fudge	1 oz	115	Resse's Cup	1 cup	92
Gum Drops	1 oz	100	Reggie Bar	1 bar	290
Hard Candy	1 oz	100	Rolo	1 thang	30
Jelly Beans	1 oz	105	Snickers	1 bar	275
Marshmallows	1 oz	90	Starburst	1 smackin	120
Mints	1 oz	100	Sugar Babies	1 baby	6
Nougats	1 oz	120	Sugar Daddy	1 sucka	121
Peanut Brittle	1 oz	120	Sugar Mamma	1 Mamma	101
Raisinettes	1 oz	120	Summit Bar	1 thang	115
Hershey Bar	1 oz	187	Turkish Taffy	1 oz	110
Baby Ruth	1 bar	260	Three Musketeers	1 thang	99
Butterfinger	1 bar	220	Tootsie Roll	1 tootsie	72
Charleston Chew	1 bar	180	World Series Bar	1 thang	130
Nestle's Crunch	1 bar	150	Zagnut	1 bar	92
Chuckles	1 bar	95			
Clark Bar	1 bar	188			
Dutch Treat	1 oz	160			
Good & Plenty	1 oz	100			
JuJubes	smidgen	15			
Hershey's Kiss	1 kiss	27			
Kit Kat	1 bar	80			
Licorice, Black	1 thang	94			
Licorice, Red	1 thang	98			

PIES

	Amt*	Cal		Amt*	Cal
Apple	1	405	Mincemeat	1	428
Banana Cream	1	335	Peach Cobbler	1	450
Blackberry	1	385	Pecan	1	595
Blueberry	1	385	Pineapple Custard	1	400
Boston Cream	1	208	Pineapple	1	365
Butterscotch	1	405	Pumpkin (white folk's)	1	321
Cherry	1	415	Pumpkin (black folk's)	1	489
Chocolate Chiffon	1	460	Raisin	1	427
Chocolate Meringue	1	355	Rhubarb	1	400
Coconut Custard	1	360	Strawberry	1	310
Lemon Meringue	1	325	Sweet Potato	1	367
Key Lime	1	300			
Egg Custard	1	310			

*Slice

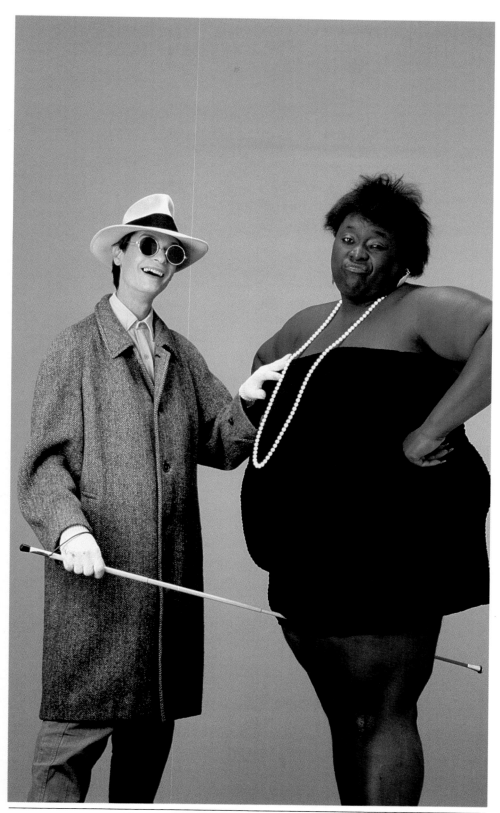

Honey, love is blind, but the scales ain't.

On behalf of us fortunate enough to have stood on
the other side of his camera,
this book is dedicated to:
KEN TOWLE
whose art was the signature of his passion
and verve.

□ ACKNOWLEDGEMENTS

Finally in a serious vein, once again I've tried to give you a bit of laughter. Laughter, perhaps that has been born out of a certain pain of being special. I still say there are no victims, only volunteers, and there are no losers, just cheaters. Ours is not to do great things or not so great things, but just to take what we have and do what we can.

So, if I've made just one smile scamper across your face, then I've done what I set out to do, and that was make your time a little bit better. Because time is the most precious resource that we have; so much more precious than we treat it, and we really should try to spend as much of it as we possibly can on smiles and laughter for they are the true treasure of this earth.

In loving memory of my niece,
Jacquelyn Kay Hollingsworth Hawthorne

Who would have written some truly wonderful things for us, if she had only had the time.